CW00524093

Intermittent Fasting for Women Over 50

The Personalized Diet Plan to Lose Belly Fat and Restore Hormone Balance Using the 16/8 Method

By

Sasha Taylor

TABLE OF CONTENTS

INTRODUCTION

Intermittent fasting, that is, periods of voluntary abstinence from food and drink, has been practised throughout the world since ancient times. The books on ethnology and religion mention a great variety of fasting forms and practices. The renewed interest in fasting is evidenced by an excess of publications and dietary recommendations of the popular press.

Dozens of books promote various forms of fasting, and hundreds of sites related to the subject can be found on the Internet. However, the scientific evidence on the health benefits of intermittent fasting in humans, often extrapolated from animal studies, is based on observational data about religious fasting (especially Ramadan) or comes from experimental studies with modest samples.

The objective of this study is to provide an overview of intermittent fasting programs and summarize the evidence about their health benefits. Because many of the data on the subject comes from research in animal models, critical studies in rodents are briefly summarized.

The results of interest in health are changes in weight and metabolic parameters associated with type 2 diabetes, cardiovascular disease, and cancer. An overview is also presented on the main mechanisms that are postulated to link fasting with human health, that is, circadian biology, the gastrointestinal microbiota, and modifiable lifestyle habits, such as food, activity, and sleep. Finally, conclusions about the evidence on intermittent fasting as an intervention to improve health are presented, and an agenda for research is proposed.

In this ebook, we will talk about intermittent fast and what you need to know about them, especially for women over 50. Enjoy!!!

CHAPTER 1
WHAT IS INTERMITTENT FASTING?

Even if fasting at intervals or intermittent fasting sounds almost outrageously novel, the opposite is the case. Like many other diets, interval fasting is a recurring phenomenon. In simple language, Interval fasting means nothing more than "interrupting" fasting in various ways. This is not a diet, such as a diet consisting of low carb or low fat, but the oldest form of nutrition that humans know.

A form of nutrition that we no longer had to practice due to sedentary life, livestock, and agriculture. In practice, it involves alternating periods of food intake and fasting. The Interval model is based on the daily routine of hunters and gatherers. After all, before the so-called Neolithic Revolution, the man spent much of the day chasing animals and collecting all kinds of berries, fruits, and nuts.

Of reality, there was no space during this period for constant food consumption, as is the case with our modern societies. The people only had time to eat food in peace when the "loot" returned to the village. Intermittent fasting is, in theory, the most efficient form of the human diet, which is especially useful due to its simplicity of execution.

11

What differentiates intermittent fasting from religious fasting and other diets?

Why don't we talk so far about a particular distribution of macronutrients or the renunciation of certain foods? Simply because at this point, the Interval quickly leaves you more or less free. It's a basic system, as I said, with simple rules that you can tailor to your individual preferences. There are no explicit rules except for an existing calorie deficit, although of course, you should eat foods that are balanced and rich in proteins. However, if you design fasting at intervals such as low carb, low fat, or high carb diet, it is up to you.

Also, for religious fasting, as practised in Islam, for example, during the fasting month of Ramadan, there are some differences. First, it is about the possibility of configuring the windows of Lent and, secondly, it is about the collection of liquid. While in Ramadan, the strict interpretation also prohibits fluid intake, with some exceptions, during intermittent fasting, you can drink as much as you want during Lenten periods. The only requirement is that it should be drunk without calories. But that should be clear.

CHAPTER 2
THE BENEFITS OF INTERMITTENT FASTING

Interstitial fasting has some critical advantages over other diets and diets. This refers, among other things, to the hormonal environment for burning fat. Who eats something every three hours, whose body is basically in the continual digestive process. The decisive starting point here is the level of blood sugar. As it does not rise gradually during the day due to the small periods for food intake, it also increases the sensitivity of insulin in the body.

At the same time, always that the release of anabolic growth hormone HGH. The conclusion is that it optimizes the biosynthesis of proteins and consumes fat. Research also shows that this diet can protect cells in the body against oxidative stress and the harmful effects of free radicals. It has also been shown that fasting cycles can lower LDL cholesterol levels by activating nerve cells and have a positive impact on cognitive performance. But the physical effects were not finished. Another advantage is the ease of implementation since you don't have to continually pay attention to specific nutritional plans or explicit food bans, as well as nutrient times. Interval fasting is an optimal form of diet if you want to eat enough despite your diet

13

or if you want to participate in celebrations or a restaurant, visit your friends without significant restrictions. All that is needed is proper time management to get the correct windows.

What are the disadvantages of intermittent fasting?

There is no perfect way of example that also applies to extended fasting. Of course, to be efficient with this system, you also need to consider certain drawbacks from the very outset. Unless you feel that you can survive without games, then you're mistaken. The fasting time is only half as adequate without strength training and supplementary endurance activities. There's nothing in here, even without a predominantly healthy diet. Occasionally junk food is permitted, but it may not be scandalous. So with that principle, you don't get a free pass to celebrate.

One of the most significant drawbacks is also on the psychological side. Mainly if you are used to eating several times a day, you should get used to not eating for many hours. Especially in the early days, the danger is particularly significant to enjoy the discomfort of the epigastrium, the so-called hunger pain. On the other hand, intermittent fasting is not suitable for people who, unfortunately, have already overcome an acute eating disorder since conversion can promote such an eating disorder. Due to the sharp decrease in blood sugar levels, the fasting interval is also not suitable for people with diabetes.

As an original form of human nutrition, fasting at intervals is not far from our internal conditioning. Consequently, the potential for weight loss success is excellent. And that the method works has already demonstrated hundreds of thousands of people. If you want to get rid of annoying body fat effectively and mentally rely on this nutritional form, then you should give a fasting interval opportunity.

CHAPTER 3
HOW TO START INTERMITTENT FASTING

The young intermittent is psychologically more affordable for the "beginners of the fast" (less deprivation) and more comfortable to implement daily in ordinary social life. It can be done over a more extended period than complete fasting because it puts the organism less at the test. There is minimal risk of suffering a "healing crisis" with intermittent fasting (signs of detoxification such as migraines, digestive disorders, nausea, etc.).

In practice, I recommend skipping dinner (or breakfast). It is simpler socially and less harsh for people who exercise a demanding professional activity. Only water (or herbal teas or broths) is allowed during the skipped meal.

Start by doing this intermittent youth once a week (e.g., Sunday morning), then gradually increase until you find your cruising pace. This type of fasting can be done all the year or by the cure of some weeks.

Of course, to reap the benefits, have the rest of the time a varied and balanced diet by limiting deli meats, red meat, dairy products, fries, pastries, and sweets! Choose raw fruits and vegetables (whole or in juice, soups), whole grains and legumes, eggs, white meats, and fish!

ALL YOU have TO KNOW BEFORE YOU START

More and more people swear by interval fasting. While some of them want to get rid of annoying pounds, others want to promote their health by fasting. We'll tell you what the trend is. Once you start fasting in this section, we'll explain what you need to know. All right, read on.

No normal fasting cure

Firstly, did you know that interval fasting and intermittent fasting are the same? Well, read on. Intermittent fasting differs in some ways from other conventional fasting methods. While with fasting practices such as Buchinger's fasting, the calorie intake is reduced over days or weeks, fasting during interval fasting often only by the hour. Normal fasting cures are usually carried out once or twice a year. Intermittent fasting, on the other hand, is used daily or at least weekly.

Normal fasting cures are often used to detoxify or detoxify the body. Such treatments are characterized by low-calorie intake and are often associated with a colon cleanse. This can be done either alone at home or in a clinic under medical supervision. These cures are supposed to free the so-called slags and the associated suffering. These methods are not suitable for losing weight.

Those who intermittently fast, on the other hand, have entirely different goals. Losing weight is often one of the main reasons because, with the interval, fasting pounds can disappear, without the metabolism suffers or even muscle mass is diminished. By regular fasting, fat metabolism is positively influenced. The metabolism learns to use its reserves because the body breaks down fat and turns it into energy. This leads to weight loss without having to follow a strict diet.

These are common methods.

Interval fasting is the generic term for many methods, all of which are characterized by a regular Lent. While some ways only last for hours, others reduce their calorie intake for up to two days. All methods should be part of everyday life, so daily or weekly, to achieve a significant effect.

The 16:8 method

The 16:8 method is probably the best-known procedure for interval fasting. Here you fast for 16 hours a day and has a time window of 8 hours to eat meals. That means you miss a meal. This can either be breakfast or dinner. If you omit breakfast, you could eat in the time window from 12 noon to

8 clocks in the evening. If you prefer to miss dinner, there is a time slot from 9 am to 5 pm.

You can generally eat in the 8 hours when meals are taken. You should not restrict your calorie intake, but do not take more than usual. Also, sugary and fatty foods are not forbidden, but a better effect can be achieved if you have a balanced and healthy diet. It's good for your health too. You should not eat for four to five hours between meals. Snacks between the main meals can lead to food cravings and interrupt fat loss. It would be better to take water or unsweetened herbal teas.

Interval fasting with the 16:8 method: instructions and example plan:

- **7 am:** Get up and drink plenty of water to keep the body hydrated. Sports on an empty stomach can increase calorie consumption and boost metabolism. But you should not overdo it. It offers short running training.
- **Morning:** Coffee is allowed during interval fasting. Fasting can, therefore, be bridged with a cup of black coffee. Tea is also available. However, drinks should be calorie-free. Sweetened beverages and latte coffee are out of the question.
- **Noon:** Fast breakage. The first meal is coming up. Since a meal is omitted daily,

you should pay attention to sufficient calorie intake. Active and healthy is a wholesome meal with vegetables, egg whites, and whole grains. When eating, you should take your time and enjoy the meal.

- **Afternoon:** You should refrain from snacks here. But you can grab tea and coffee again. After 16 o'clock, however, one should better abstain from caffeine so as not to impair the sleep rhythm.
- **19 o'clock:** Last meal of the day. Again, you should go back to a balanced meal. A dessert is also allowed. For a fruit salad or quark offers. For dinner, you can drink a glass of wine or a beer, but alcohol should only be consumed in small quantities.
- **Evening:** At 20 o'clock begins the fasting. Now only water and caffeine-free teas should be consumed. Eight hours of sleep a day provide rest. So you can sleep half the time of Lent.

The 5: 2 method

Instead of fasting daily, Lent is limited to two days a week. Five days a week, you can eat healthy meals and do not have to spend time. Food intake is significantly reduced over the remaining two days. Women consume only 500 calories per day;

Men eat 600 calories a day. Carbohydrates are entirely dispensed with. Instead, one resorts to vegetable broths, vegetables, and protein-containing foods. This method works best if you always fast on the same days of the week. This is especially the weekend. Since the calorie intake is significantly reduced, you should plan sufficient rest periods and less strenuous activities.

Alternating fasting

Alternating fasting is made up of a typical day and a fasting day that always alternate. Another name for this method is "10 in 2". It stands for the one day you eat (1) and the fast day (0), which together make two days (2). Discipline is required here because the calorie intake is significantly reduced on the fasting day. While you do not have to pay attention to your diet for one day, the following day, you only eat vegetable broths, water, and unsweetened teas. When feasting, you should not only resort to sugary and fatty foods. A balanced diet is essential so that the body receives all the necessary nutrients.

Alternatives: fast for 12 hours or one day a week

If these methods are too strict and still want to try interval fasting, Shorten the fasting time a little bit. Instead of fasting for 16 hours a day, you can start with 12 hours. Here one slept most of the Lent and

21

has to sleep for eight hours with only four hours without a meal. A suitable time window would be, for example, a Lent from 8 pm to 8 am. So you have to do without dinner or breakfast.

If you prefer to fast every week instead of daily, you can start on a fasting day. Here you fast for 24 hours and feeds exclusively on vegetable broths, water, teas, and juices. You should refrain from solid food. Fasting can be started either for breakfast, lunch, or dinner. There must be 24 consecutive hours.

Which is the best for women over 50?

Be aware of this:

Partial fasting affects the female hormone balance.

Therefore women over 50, in particular, should fast carefully. It is quite possible that women feel uncomfortable and tired during fasting.

Other women report that they are on the 16/8 diet

- Had no hot flashes at night.
- Are much more balanced.
- Would have slept through.
- No longer had a racing heart at night.

If you are not sure whether interval fasting is suitable for you, you should consult your doctor.

Note:

- Do not fast on consecutive days. Instead, fast, for example, Tuesday, Thursday and Saturday.
- Do not fast for more than 12 to 13 hours. A fasting phase between 7 p.m. and 8 a.m. is ideal, for example. With a longer fasting window, a stress reaction is triggered
- Do not train too hard on fasting days. Instead of intense exercises like HIIT, long runs or strength training you should on yoga or light cardio training set
- Make sure you drink enough water when you fast
- Your diet should be tailored to your hormonal needs and contain little flammable substances. That means: no gluten, no sugar, no dairy or red meat
- Very important: listen to your body. If you are not feeling well at fasting, have a headache or are irritable, do not overdo it. Every woman reacts differently to not eating. Be careful with yourself and take it easy on the days you fast.

CHAPTER 4
MYTHS ABOUT INTERMITTENT FASTING

On fasting, many myths continue to be disseminated even by health professionals. Here are five of those myths that you must stop believing in taking advantage of the benefits of this nutritional approach.

Along with the ketogenic diet, the use of fasting as a nutritional and dietary intervention has become popular in recent years. Practical and scientific reasons are not lacking, as we have already discussed in other articles; like the fact that for many cases, a controlled fasting regime is better than simply adopting one of many popular diets.

However, much information that we know today is wrong continues to be disseminated even by health professionals who do not end up getting rid of conceptions promoted for decades and that became nutritional dogma. For example, we need to eat three times a day.

But here we have, backed by serious scientific studies, most carried out in recent decades, five of the most widespread myths totally wrong about fasting, a style of food that is actually neither new nor dangerous.

24

And if it's a fad, it has been for hundreds of thousands of years.

1. Skipping breakfast makes you fat

The myth that continues to spread as done by nutritionists. The idea that breakfast is the most important meal of the day is only true when the daily diet is (badly) based on carbohydrates.

Studies have already shown that overweight and obese people showed no difference in weight in 16 weeks, whether they ate breakfast or not. In fact, other studies suggest that the opposite is true: those who lose weight in the long term are those who usually eat breakfast.

Obviously, what you eat and when you eat the rest of the meals of the day influences your metabolism, but in general, it is a good practice not to have breakfast until you actually starve yourself.

In addition, skipping breakfast will only make you fat if what you eat later will be foods high in calories and low in healthy fats, protein and micronutrients, such as flours, pasta and sugars.

So don't blame the fact of not having breakfast, but the poor nutritional quality of what you eat.

2. Eating frequently improves your metabolism, reduces appetite, helps you lose weight and is good for your health

As we can see by the increase in cases of obesity, diabetes and all other members of the Metabolic Syndrome in recent decades, eating three or more times a day is not the solution to achieve a healthy weight.

Contrary, again, to what the traditional professional council says, we do not need to eat three times a day. This advice comes from a custom that only exists since the industrial revolution when working hours made it necessary to establish schedules for food.

Eating frequently, recent studies prove, in fact, it promotes the storage of calories in the form of fat, which over time encourages diabetes and many other chronic conditions related to excess calories.

In other words, eating more times a day does not increase the metabolic rate, nor reduce hunger, much less help you lose weight. What it does is the nutrient composition of what you eat and the time you give your body to manage these calories metabolically.

3. Your brain needs a regular intake of food glucose

Another great myth is a product of the comfort provided by the food industry in the last 100 years and not a fact-based on the metabolic functioning of the human body.

To date, the nutritional standard continues to consider the consumption of carbohydrates in the composition of food necessary because "carbohydrates provide energy". And they do it. But that energy is useful only in the short term. Carbohydrates are basically cheap fuel and easy to burn. But also to store. And it is not essential.

The human body can easily produce more and better energy from fats. In addition, human metabolism evolved to be able to synthesize the glucose necessary for the brain and other tissues of other macronutrients such as lipids and proteins. So we don't need carbohydrates from food directly. And much less refined carbohydrates.

In fact, we now know what the Inuit and all our ancestors before the adoption of agriculture took advantage of: the human body, including the brain, works best in a state of ketosis, that is, with fat as its primary source of energy, and no carbohydrates

4. Fasting puts your body in starvation mode and makes you lose muscle

As we discussed in an earlier article , it is an urban legend that muscle is lost only by fasting. In fact, as we also summarize, combining exercise and fasting is better for many reasons.

However, we do not stop listening to the advice of eating before exercising, and that fasting encourages the famous state of starvation. According to this myth, if we don't eat for several hours or days, our body will eat itself, and the muscle will degrade when the opposite is what happens.

We now know from various studies that the fasting state, in fact, encourages the work of hormones that promote not only muscle preservation but also their development. If this myth of the "starvation mode" were true, the human race would have long since died out in one of many seasons of food shortages.

As Dr Jason Fung explains in many of his talks on the subject, "the body is not stupid" and evolved to consume muscle proteins only as a last resort, precisely because muscle is what it takes to move in search of food.

5. Fasting makes you overeat

Clear. But only when it is your habit to feed yourself with meals of very little nutritional value.

It is obvious that when what we eat are calories that are saved or burned quickly, if we wait several hours to eat, we will tend to eat much more than necessary. However, as in the case of muscle that is preserved and even gained, fasting by eating the right foods, in fact, will help you need less food to function not only the same but better.

Once the adaptation time has passed (which differs depending on your eating and genetic habits), fasting for a longer time will be easier, and not vice versa, as many people, including health professionals, still believe.

It's that simple: several studies have already proven that fasting reduces insulin levels, increases metabolic rate (the rate at which you burn calories), norepinephrine and growth hormone levels; What makes you lose fat, don't gain it .

And this is why intermittent fasting is becoming as famous as an intervention to lose weight and combat conditions such as diabetes.

How to take advantage of the benefits of fasting?

Fasting, as we saw in relation to all these myths, brings many benefits for metabolism and health in general, among them and very importantly, the activation of what is considered a system of self-protection of the body that evolved to survive; but that now we can take advantage to live more and with greater health.

But this is the subject of the following article on intermittent fasting, the most practical technique to integrate fasting into our diet and take advantage of all the advantages of emulating the way our ancestors fed for hundreds of thousands of years.

CHAPTER 5
WHEN SHOULD YOU AVOID INTERMITTENT FASTING?

Intermittent fasting has proven to be an effective and interesting method to help in the fight against overweight. However, it is not always convenient to get carried away by the fame that this nutritional pattern is taking. And, in some cases, intermittent fasting could prove harmful. What cases are we talking about?

As we have spoken on numerous occasions, intermittent fasting is an interesting and effective method of promoting fat consumption and weight loss. Of course, it is no miracle system, and its effects may not be noticed immediately, which does not mean that scientific evidence has shown that this system has long-term benefits.

In particular, fasting for 12 or 20 hours in a row can reduce the risk factors for cardiovascular and metabolic diseases, or even reverse some of its consequences. A lower incidence of cancer and neurodegenerative diseases has also been found among practitioners of this pattern. Although we do not know for sure what are the mechanisms that act after this, it is probably based on our circadian rhythms .

These control the metabolism by segregating melatonin and a cascade of signals that stimulate our body. If we consider it from the evolutionary point of view, the circadian rhythm is better adapted for thousands of years of evolution to fasting. But before embarking on practising it, we must bear in mind that intermittent fasting should not be practised by all people at all costs.

When should intermittent fasting not be practised?

It must be made clear that, outside of these cases, intermittent fasting (and fasting in general) has not shown any problem or harm. Moreover, we insist, it has been shown to have an important series of benefits: blood glucose level control, cardiovascular problem control, cancer prevention... However, it is better to take care of yourself in the following cases:

When you need a lot of energy

Not all bodies work the same, nor do all bodies need the same amount of energy. If we need a large number of calories, intermittent fasting is completely contraindicated. What occasions do we mean? Normally in the case of being underweight (with a BMI below 18.5).

The latter is important because the body is a machine to consume energy, and it is also growing. If someone under the age of 18 decides to perform this dietary pattern, it is important that you consult a doctor or a professional dietitian-nutritionist first. It is also totally out of place when there is an eating disorder, such as anorexia or bulimia, obviously.

When we suffer from sleep problems

Intermittent fasting, especially when you start your practice, can change many of our habits. That includes our dream, which can be affected in a very unpleasant way. The change of pattern has important metabolic consequences. If we suffer from insomnia or similar problems, it is better that we avoid intermittent fasting. In short, the benefit that we will obtain will not be compensated by the problems that will give us the worst sleep.

When we have anxiety problems, stress...

As with sleep, if we suffer from stress or anxiety, it is better to leave intermittent fasting aside. Changing our metabolic pattern is expensive at the mood level , and our mood will suffer a lot. The fault lies, again, with our metabolism, which increases the levels of hormones that signal alertness, and makes us more aggressive and predisposed to depression.

In addition, anxious behaviours can translate into something else: compulsive eating. This happens many more times than it seems. As we have said other times, the period of intake of intermittent fasting is not equal to a white letter from the binge, in which we can eat everything we want and how much we want. Food must follow a healthy and adequate pattern. Eating compulsively, in these cases (and in any other), goes against the ultimate goal and "the remedy can be worse than the disease."

When there are metabolic problems

In the case of suffering from high uric acid problems, metabolic syndrome or even diabetes , intermittent fasting is discouraged. Actually, it is not that it cannot be practised, but, at the very least, we should consult with a specialist who tells us what we should do and how we should do it . This way we will avoid serious problems and unpleasant surprises that could end very badly.

This, roughly, is due to the metabolic change that drives intermittent fasting. Used to living in a constant cycle of intake, all metabolism will be pressured to change our blood glucose levels, fat mobilization, changes in the cascade of hormones and signals ... in this very complex process we could jeopardize some important step for our health . If we suffer from a disease, it is best to inform ourselves well and by a specialist before embarking on the adventure of fasting.

CHAPTER 6

HOW CAN I LOSE SOME WEIGHT IN A MONTH

Rapid Yet Sustained Weight Loss

One month, one stone, one concerted effort

Let's figure out what's necessary to achieve this. If we believe we will lose about 5lbs every 10 days for 30 days per month (Approximately 2 kg or 15 lb in 3 days or 0.5lb / day or more than 3lbs per week).

I'll take an imaginary man and woman and put down some figures for them. Tell yourself how to do it if you're different from my examples.

If we conclude that there are about 3500 calories in a pound of fat, so if you want to get those 3lbs off (3500x 14lbs= 49000cals), you need to build a deficit of at least 11500 calories every week.

It's a daily deficit of about 1,600 calories if we break that down into every day.

Now, let's find out how much energy remaining alive costs:

I'll take three men and three women.

Male 1

- 70kg -11st 0.3lb - 154.3lbs
- Cals (range) of energy 1,918-3,036

Male 2

- 80 kg — 12th 8.4 lb — 176.4lbs
- Power calcium 2.038-3.226.

Male 3

- 90 kg-14th 2.4 lb-198.4lbs
- Energy range 2,158-3,416 Cals.

Female 1

- 60 kg — 9th 6.3 lb — 132.3lbs
- Power level 1,598-2,531

Female 2

- 70kg -11st 0.3lb - 154.3lbs
- Cals (range) of energy-1,718-2,721

Female 3

- 80 kg-12th 8.4 lb-176.4lbs
- Energy-1,838-2,911 Cals (range)

Notes: The ranges for daily calorie expenditure depend on the activity level, from sedentary (think office worker who drives to work and takes no or very limited exercise) to highly active (someone with a job involving several hours of manual work per day or exercises at a high intensity / consistently high heart rate per day for more than 90 minutes).

These fictional figures are based on someone in their mid-30s, who is about 170 cm tall. They are used for illustration purposes only, the principles behind the practices here are valid, you need to personalize the practices to your situation.These are averages only and will vary from person to person; you need to get your starting figures to find out more accurately. You can use the calculators found on caloriesperhour.com to do this. For a rough starting point, use the BMR and RMR calcs, then use the techniques here to change the figures based on the results of the real world. For a 60 kg woman, who is only mildly active or sedentary!

So you can see that this would mean no eating at all for about a month

For whom is this? Nonetheless, a 60 kg woman doesn't have to lose 14lbs (about 6 kg) or more than 10% of her body weight, so we don't have to care for that individual. The upper end of the scale is what we should look for. That's where the large numbers of weight loss are very realistic.

If you look at the 90 kg man, for example, even a

sedentary person could cut off more than 1000 cals from their daily intake, as long as they do it with the right foods. In a second, I'm going to come to that.

First, Let's look briefly at the three factors that will allow for this significant calorie reduction.

1: Intermittent Fasting

Intermittent fasting (the version of Leangains) is a simple way to feed the body. You divide the day into two phases, a phase of eating and a phase of eating. It takes about 8 hours to eat. The fasting period thus lasts roughly 16 hours. This doesn't mean you're eating the whole8-hour block!

There are two key aspects to Intermittent Fasting that make massive weight loss work for you.

1: Physiologically, every day is divided into two distinct phases, each of which helps your fat loss goal. These two phases are an anabolic, or tissue-building phase, and a fat-burning, or energy breakdown phase.

2: Using IF makes it much easier than traditional diets to reduce your calories

You should definitely do some sort of IF if you want to make your weight loss as painless and effective as possible.

2: Food high, low-fat, low-carbon

In his excellent series of posts on developing a diet for fat loss, Lyle MacDonald is talking about setting it up from the ground instead of from the top. What are you saying? Okay, what we've done here is to start with a target of weight loss, which is the top or limit, and then work backwards to find out what we need to do. Lyle takes a slightly different approach in those papers and works out what you need physiologically, and then brings those figures into a diet to see what ends up coming out. Here we will use part of that strategy (setting protein intake) to give you a starting point for finding out what you are eating.

How much food do you need?

And, more precisely, how much protein to each meal will you strive for? Well, we can answer this question in two ways, the best answer is the one that makes you feel most reassured. The quick answer is' lots.' The more precise response is worked out as follows; begin with a bodyweight level of about 1g / lb and break over your two or three meals, then change based on lean tissue and decreases in strength and levels of hunger / satiety. So if you find your strength falling and your muscle leaving your body, you need to add more protein to it, and if you feel hungry between meals or you are not happy with a meal, add more protein!

What Foods Can I Eat?

One thing I consistently find on this type of diet is the total lack of appetite and feelings of deprivation, and this should not be shocking given the enormous range of foods on offer here. One thing you will notice is the total lack of powders / protein drinks for liquid foods / meal substitution. This is deliberate; they do not provide satiety and fulfilment, and they provide no incentive for long-term adherence to the diet. "Don't drink your calories," as Martin Berkhan says.

Why High Protein, Low Fat, Low Carb?

A few reasons; 1, you want the calories to be kept as low as possible, as easily as possible. 2, Protein plus lots of bulky yet low-carbon foods make it easy to feel full, satisfied, and happy when you cut calories.

3: Doing only high-intensity weights and very low-intensity cardio

Each of the three elements is equally important in this weight loss plan, so you'd better find a way of including this part! Just ask yourself if it's worth jeopardizing the whole plan for the sake of missing some simple exercises?

Why start with a statement like that?

Since slipping back into old ways of ' training for weight loss ' is too easy for many people.

What you need to do is heavyweights, with low reps and using as big as possible movements. Remember, large weights are totally specific to each individual, and the actual number / weight is irrelevant; what is important is that you lift up to YOUR ability and learn how to lift fully at your ability. This means learning what a max effort lift feels like AND expecting the max to go up quickly while you know how to get more and more out of yourself for those of you who have hardly lifted weights before.

This program's great thing about it is that it is easy. Take and repeat the following exercises:

- Squat
- Dumbell press, bench press or bodyweight dips
- Dumbell or barbell shoulder press
- Lat pull-down, pull-up, sitting row, or bent over Deadlift barbell / dumbell
- track.

Your rotation is easy: Do 5set 4-6 reps for 3 weeks (routine 5x5 style) and then 3 weeks of 9-12 reps (routine 3x10 style). You increase the weight every time you hit the upper rep range. You only have to rest after 10-14 weeks (but if you've regularly been training for more than twelve weeks, you need to take a week of complete rest right now-unless you're planning within 12 weeks from the beginning of your plan, in which case you'll get your rest at the end!)

If you don't know how these exercises can be done, you can get instructions from a competent trainer (you can find out if they're good by watching how they get you to move and focus on your learning exercises if they get you to do your exercises like those done in instruction videos you're probably sure they know their stuff), or you can check out the abundance of vids on YouTube and figure out your way.

CHAPTER 7
HOW THE WOMAN'S BODY CHANGES

The body does not stop changing throughout our lives. Age and genetics are primarily responsible for these changes, although not the only ones. External factors such as tobacco, alcohol, poor diet or excessive sunbathing are determinants for the deterioration of our health over the decades.

In the case of women, the amount of hormones that we have determines the evolution of our body over the decades. Fertility is also key to understanding the changes that occur. "Between the decades of the 20s and 60s, the woman undergoes a series of important changes, both hormonally and physically, as a result of menstrual cycles, pregnancies and other derivatives of reproductive ageing.

At 20 years old

During this decade, the woman is full of energy and performance and we enjoy a baseline health status. The body adapts to our rhythm of life and we perform better physically.

Genetics is a fundamental factor that determines endogenous ageing, however, everything takes its toll. As much as at 20 years the skin is full of collagen, a weekend of excesses on the beach or smoking daily are points that accumulate against the epidermis and time. "If a person with a genetic predisposition to have a thinner dermis or lighter skin, also smokes, sunbathes and excessive gesticulation, may have wrinkles in the 20s.

Creating good eating and exercise habits while avoiding alcohol and smoking, as well as paying attention to eating disorders and attending gynaecological exams annually.

As for the skin, during this decade and the third, the woman loses the brightness of adolescence and therefore must start using moisturizers, which should subsequently be rich in alpha-hydroxy acids.

During the second decade, the woman is in the fullness of her sexual development by ovarian activity. The secretion of hormones such as estrogen and progesterone play a fundamental role in the menstrual cycle and fertility.

At birth, our ovaries have a million oocytes and will no longer be produced. In each menstrual cycle, they are discarded, so as time progresses the possibility of becoming a mother decreases until menopause arrives. Between the ages of 15 and 25, the probability of becoming pregnant in each cycle is 40 per cent. During this time, contraceptive treatments should be taken into account to avoid unwanted pregnancy as well as assistance in the transmission of infectious diseases.

At 30

From the age of 30, there is a decrease in metabolism, which means that, if we do not exercise, we burn fewer calories per minute naturally.

The specialist Concepción de Lucas points out that if you also lead a sedentary lifestyle, with work stress or poor diet, our physical condition can get worse.

In addition, this is the decade in which most Spanish women have their first child: the average is 32 years old. The expert points out that this moment is key for women. "In this decade, muscle tone is lost and, with pregnancy, the body can undergo significant changes, with increases and decreases in weight, body volume and muscle sagging."

It is also common to observe adult acne, which usually appears in the jaw area and that is due to an excessive sensitivity of the skin of that area to hormonal changes and that can be treated with oral contraceptive treatments or oral recurrences (not indicated for pregnant women since it can cause alteration is in the fetus) or synthetic, as dermatologist María Teresa Truchuelo explains. This type of acne may also be due to disorders such as the polycystic ovary or the use of overly fatty cosmetics.

From the age of 30, expression wrinkles begin to appear in the areas where we are most gesturing, such as between the eyebrows or the eye area, with bags and crow's feet. The specialist recommends using moisturizers and containing active ingredients such as the aforementioned alpha hydroxy acids, which seek to reshape the skin, vitamin C and niacinamide.

You have to maintain good eating and exercise habits, go to gynaecological exams annually and do health checks to monitor cholesterol, weight, visual and auditory acuity and the early detection of diseases and pathologies.

From the age of 35, the woman's fertility decreases and it is increasingly difficult to get pregnant, so gynaecologists advise not to delay motherhood beyond this age because, in addition to having to resort to assisted reproduction techniques, They add the risks of having abortions, hypertension, diabetes and deformations or alterations in the fetus. From the age of 40, the probability of pregnancy in each cycle is 25 per cent.

At 40

During the fourth decade of our life, a series of changes in our physiognomy begin to occur. The fat that predominated in the buttocks and legs for possible breastfeeding begins to redistribute in the abdomen, increasing the risk of cardiovascular disease.

Also, decrease muscle mass and tone and increases sagging in arms and legs, especially if we do not exercise.

The level of hormones drops and the woman is moving away from her period of greatest fertility.

The skin loses elasticity and sunspots begin to develop like antigens, which are more marked on the lighter skins. "Expression wrinkles intensify, and facial volumes begin to vary. The expert recommends anti-spot lasers, botulinum toxin for expression wrinkles and hyaluronic acid to treat wrinkles of the nasogenial groove and volume loss.

Good eating habits and exercise will contribute to a better menopausal transition in the future, as Lucas warns. The specialist indicates that, from the age of 40, the tendency to suffer from hypertension and cholesterol, pathologies that are also observed in men, rises.

In addition, the intervertebral discs are compressed, and it is normal for spine pain, loss of muscle tone to increase and osteoporosis or loss of bone mass. "It is important that young women prevent their appearance by performing a diet rich in calcium and muscle strength exercises. This serves to condition the muscles, make them stronger and stronger. It also strengthens the union of muscle with a bone through tendons.

From 45-50 years old, women can begin to notice hot flashes, irritability, difficulty sleeping, vaginal dryness, decreased libido and alterations in menstruation; We are in premenopause, " explains Esparza, who advises seeing it as" a natural stage in women, "which must be normalized and treated if necessary to reduce symptoms. "We must not fear it, or there are methods to prevent it, simply accept it as another stage as a person and as a woman.

From the age of 45, early menopause can also occur, which usually occurs between 50 and 55 years.

From 50 years old

During the 50s, women begin to suffer from menopause, which is the absence of menstruation for more than 12 months and is due to the permanent cessation of follicular function. Its diagnosis is clinical and retrospective when 12 months have elapsed since the last period without any menstrual bleeding.

Lucas's conception clarifies that "there are no clear guidelines on how to deal with it because each woman has different experiences, but most of the changes in their bodies are related to it."

During this period, the alteration in the distribution of body fat continues, the appearance of the skin in terms of elasticity and hydration worsens, vaginal dryness and other mucous membranes that can cause pain during sexual intercourse are experienced, muscle tone decreases and muscle damage deteriorates. Bones of the spine, joints or osteoarthritis problems appear.

"It also increases cardiovascular risk, sleep and memory disorders influenced by the gradual loss of estrogen," explains the specialist, adding that changes in lifestyle can cause several changes in mood: " during this stage, it is normal to suffer more anxiety, depression and a decrease in mood. "

The woman who is in the fifth decade may also notice that she loses pubic and axillary hair, undergoes changes in hair and skin or increases in body weight.

Menopause causes that, between 50 and 60 years, the woman's skin experiences many alterations. "The decrease in estrogen that occurs at this time in the woman's life leads to a thinning of the skin and dehydration, which causes wrinkles to intensify and 'sagging' of structures.

Acclimatizing the body to the symptoms of menopause by reducing body temperature with light clothing and drinking cold drinks, as well as exercising regularly to prevent osteoporosis. Proper nutrition, doing controlled breathing exercises and going to gynaecological exams and other medical check-ups are also tips to keep in mind during this stage and during the sixth decade of our life.

The specialist also recalls that "throughout the woman's life, the gynaecologist must be present, adapting her actions to the different health and reproductive status.

At every stage of the woman, physical changes, as well as psychological changes, occur and that the specialist must be a foothold to ask constantly. " These are vital phases that must be accepted and lived. Every change you don't understand or doubt you have, you will have your gynaecologist to solve them.

CHAPTER 8
IMPLEMENTATION OF PHYSICAL ACTIVITY

The incorporation into the daily routine of a constant and moderate physical activity induces a series of physiological changes in the organism that go beyond the fact of burning calories, reducing fat and maintaining muscle mass. In addition to promoting weight loss and improving the relationship with food and the body itself, physical activity induces a change in the composition of the body and the functioning of metabolism and systems (circulatory, respiratory, etc.).

Daily physical exercise, for example, is a way to improve cardiovascular health because it acts on different fronts:

- It reduces blood pressure, favouring the control of hypertension.
- Increases the secretion of HDL cholesterol (good cholesterol), reducing the rate of blood cholesterol.
- It induces a decrease in triglyceride levels.

It decreases the production of insulin, helping to control type 2 diabetes and favouring the assimilation of nutrients and their arrival in the cells of the different tissues, in addition to reducing the uptake and accumulation of fat.

physical activity

Control of cardiovascular risk factors (hypercholesterolemia, arterial hypertension and type 2 diabetes).

- Increased lung capacity.
- Increase in muscle strength and mass.
- Increase in aerobic capacity.
- Reduction of fat mass.

It improves the psychological balance of the person by inducing a state of personal satisfaction and the control of anxiety and stress.

Finally, it is worth highlighting the last benefit of physical activity and that is that it improves the individual's relationship with food, reducing appetite and favouring the adoption of healthy eating habits.

Conditions Of Use Of The Service

In no way can the information provided by this tool replace a direct health care provider, nor should it be used to determine a diagnosis, or to choose a procedure in particular cases.

No recommendation on drugs, techniques, products, etc. will be made in this service, explicitly or implicitly. That will be cited for informational purposes only. The use of this service is carried out under the exclusive responsibility of the users. The information exchanged with this service is confidential. However, its content may be published omitting any reference to personal data.

What Are The Types Of Exercises That Are The Best For You (Woman Over 50)?

It is time to set the table, but the exercises from 50 should be to get a healthy body, the following exercises work several muscles in your body as well as the buttocks and hamstrings for women over 50, create more legs stronger, thinner and with more force, to lift its rear part, the quadriceps also work, since they require that the knee be straightened with resistance.

To perform the first of these exercises, stand in front of a bench or a firm chair, place your left foot firmly on top of the bench or chair, press your left foot and push the body back until the left leg is straight, lower the body down until the right knee is flexed and repeated 10 to 15 times.

Weight balanced evenly, don't lean too far forward or too far back.

The so-called bridge exercises are not only the perfect exercise for a perfectly rounded back, but it will also help women keep their back healthy and pain-free.

Define Abs for women

To do this great exercise called a bridge, lie down with your mouth up while on the floor, with your knees slightly bent and with your feet flat on the floor, raise your hips so that your body shapes will take a curved line from the shoulders to the knees, pause in the upper position for two or three seconds, then lower your body back to the initial position, repeat this movement 10 to 15 times, then take a short rest of five minutes maximum and repeat the number of times before recommended.

Routine abdominals for women

With the addition of raising an arm while performing the previous exercise on the floor improves the posture and the strength of the base, which makes me feel better, it will seem more effort, but you will feel more secure.

Given the situation of reducing our belly, it is important to perform the exercises in a constant and linear way; it is advisable to expand the abdominal table for women in a progressive manner, every 10 or 15 days would be correct because each time we will have the most strengthened abdominal area.

Strengthen Buttocks

To perform the following exercise for women over 50 to create stronger, stronger legs and buttocks, start by adopting an iron position, but bend your elbows and lean on your forearms instead of on your hands.

Exercise table for the buttocks

Your body should create a straight line to the ankles from the shoulders, tighten your buttocks and maintain your hip position while raising your right arm forward, move your shoulder blades down and back as you raise your arms, keep the position for 5 to 10 seconds relax the buttocks and repeat the exercise ten to fifteen times changing arm.

There are so many physical and mental benefits with yoga , with the investment postures that are excellent to help reduce the appearance of cellulite, make a shoulder support or put your legs above the wall for 5 minutes every night before going to bed, this will be beneficial not only for the appearance of cellulite but also to collaborate with its circulation greatly.

Exercises for women over 50 years create stronger, thinner and stronger legs

To correctly perform the following exercise after 50, you have to take it more calmly, to create stronger, more firm legs and buttocks, lie on your back and gradually lift your hips and legs off the floor, bringing your legs they will be above your head until your toes touch the ground behind you, place your hands behind your back and extend your legs stretching them in the air, creating a straight line from your shoulders to your ankles.

Keep your neck relaxed as well as your shoulder support hold, try to hold the position for at least one minute and then slowly reach the starting position, pause, rest and then repeat the movement about ten more times, obviously with your respective breaks.

For a quick toning of the whole body, go through the movements described above and perform three sets of each of the exercises about ten times or otherwise indicated by a medical condition, move as quickly as possible between the movements to The maximum calorie intake.

The next day, do other exercises, you can incorporate a few series of cardio intervals at the time of training your entire body, or you can do it separately over a longer period of time in these exercises for women over 50 years.

If you want to reinforce a specific area, choose the exercises that focus on those places and incorporate them into your daily routine, just remember that to continue challenging your body, you should gradually increase the amount of repetitions in the proportion that get stronger.

An exercise routine for women over 50

Multidirectional exercises help develop coordination and control while providing toning and hardening of the quadriceps, buttocks, hamstrings and inner thighs.

Exercises after 50 will help keep your back healthy and pain-free

To perform the following exercise, stand with your feet together, both arms stretched over your head, palms facing forward, take a wide step with your right foot towards the corner of the room at a 45-degree angle at diagonally, bending the right knee and reaching the lower part of your body in a forward motion on your right thigh, the back leg should be straight, with your heel lifted off the floor.

Leg and buttock exercises

If you can touch the ground, do it on both sides of your right foot, lightly with your fingers, push with your right foot to return to the starting position, repeat 15 times on one leg and 15 times for the other, an option to modify. This exercise is not to go so low in the stride and aim to reach with your hands at the knee or the level of the shin instead.

Leg exercises for women

As quick advice, stand again out of the position described above and focus on working out the abdominals with tight buttocks, squeezing your thighs together and maintaining good posture.

In addition to getting thinner and stronger legs, the postures that we must adapt to maintain a healthy and erect back. In addition to hardening our legs our day to day will have a better quality of life, now I remember what it cost to climb the stairs with a smile from ear to ear.

CHAPTER 9

HOW TO USE PSYCHOLOGY TO PURSUE THE DIET CONSTANTLY AND IN THE RIGHT WAY

What we eat not only affects how we feel but also how we feel affects our way of eating.

It is for this reason that there is a branch of psychology specialized in caring for the way we feed ourselves. It is usually called Nutrition, Psychology, or Food Psychology.

Psychology and food: a tandem necessary for our health

Although many people do not believe it, psychology can be an important one to improve adherence to a diet, either to improve body image or to control excessive food intake in cases of overweight, as there are psychological variables related to success when it comes to following a diet.

Therefore, psychologists are professionals who can provide their services so that individuals can make behavioural changes or changes in lifestyle. There are tools (such as good planning, stimulus avoidance, etc.) that can be beneficial to carry out a successful dietary plan.

A psychologist can be a great help in the fight against obesity because the emotional aspects are very important when it comes to achieving a permanent change in the habits that affect food. In addition, in severe cases of eating disorders, the psychologist is an indispensable figure for the correct treatment of pathologies.

Eating with the palate: a pleasant behaviour

Many people do not eat according to their nutritional needs, but it is the palate that motivates them to eat food without control. This may seem like an everyday activity, but it can be very harmful to health if foods with a low nutritional value and a high content of substances harmful to the body (such as trans fats) are abused.

Abusing the pleasant act of eating can not only make us feel more tired and constantly look for more food, but it can cause serious health problems. Eating with the palate is a behaviour that has to do with pleasure and, therefore, the reward system, mediated by dopamine, comes into play. Dopamine is a neurotransmitter that actively participates in the reinforcement of pleasant behaviours such as sex or drug use.

Emotions affect our diet: emotional eating

On many occasions people know food pedagogy

very well, the problem is that they do not adhere to a dietary plan for many reasons: lack of motivation, unrealistic goals, negative self-efficacy beliefs, exposure to interfering stimuli and, above all, a low mood.

The emotions-nutrition relationship is clear since, in moments of emotional instability, we are more likely to consume fatty foods. This is not positive for weight control and causes excess fat in the diet. When we use the diet to calm our emotional state, this is called emotional feeding.

The psychological and emotional variables are very important to succeed in the diet since for many people, it is not an easy path. On the other hand, we must understand human behaviour and know that when we are anxious or have emotional problems, many individuals respond with large food intakes. In addition, stress also causes mood problems that influence food intake.

Depression and binge eating

In severe cases such as depression, depressed individuals often increase their food intake disproportionately. According to the Diagnostic and Statistical Manual of Mental Disorders (DSM IV) in the course of depression, episodes of overstating may occur, but without loss of control (something that does occur in binge eating disorder).

The reason why individuals with depression or emotional problems often go in search of food to feel better and calm their mood is that many foods include tryptophan, an amino acid that causes the release of serotonin (low levels of serotonin they are associated with depression and obsession).

The lack of serotonin causes different negative effects on the organism, such as anxiety, sadness or irritability. Since the body does not produce tryptophan, it must be achieved from the diet. Therefore, foods rich in this amino acid act as natural antidepressants.

There are several studies that relate serotonin with a greater sense of well-being, relaxation, better sleep, higher self-esteem, greater concentration and a better mood. In addition, serotonin has an important function of the brain because it establishes the balance between other neurotransmitters such as dopamine or norepinephrine (norepinephrine). These neurotransmitters are important as they are related to anxiety, anxiety or eating disorders.

Foods to improve our well-being

Below is a list of foods rich in Tryptophan:

- Turkey
- Chicken

- Milk
- Cheese
- Fish
- Eggs
- Tofu
- Soy
- Walnuts
- Chocolate
- Chia seeds

Finally, regarding serotonin, low levels of this neurotransmitter are associated with obsessive behaviours and binge eating disorder.

In a study published in the Journal of Clinical Investigation, he explains that researchers at the USDA / ARS Child Nutrition Research Center at Baylor College of Medicine in Houston and the Texas Children's Hospital in the United States showed that the Estrogen hormone could increase serotonin production to inhibit binge eating.

Psychology applied to nutrition

As we have commented, there is a relationship between psychology and nutrition. The so-called "Nutrition Psychology" deals with the study and application of these phenomena both in their normal conditions and in those that occur in the pathology. The quality of the link between psychism, social, emotional and educational factors, and nutrition, are essential for the healthy development of any person.

In the western world, and due to the existing socio-economic system, we have been educated to consume aesthetics. This causes pathologies or disorders of eating behaviour such as Anorexia or Bulimia if you do not work to minimize the effects of image culture. This need for exchange between disciplines such as Nutrition and Mental Health makes necessary the contribution of psychology for the healthy development of individuals.

For example, the problem of obesity is not only about losing weight; in many cases, there are certain aspects involved that must be addressed and that not only have to do with food. An individual who has been obese since childhood has never had a representation of his slim body. Any changes that occur will not only affect your weight but will have consequences on your identity. Psychology, therefore, plays an important role in people's well-being, and nutrition is an important aspect for the full development of an individual.

CHAPTER 10
INTERMITTENT FASTING AND KETOGENIC DIET

The combination of a ketogenic diet and interval fasting is said to help you lose weight - but is it really healthy?

A diet is a challenge; in the long run, requires a lot of discipline and perseverance to counter the dreaded yo-yo effect. So how can it work to combine two reduced diets? Is this possible? And how healthy is it for the body? These questions arise from the interaction of the ketogenic diet and interval fasting; both recognized ways of losing weight. But the simultaneous implementation is a different level that promises quick and effective weight loss, but also puts your own body awareness to the test. Here, the game is played with the so-called ketosis - a metabolic reaction that can be triggered with a changed diet and can outwit the body's own processes for one's own benefit.

How to combine interval fasting with the keto diet?

When it comes to trendy foods, interval fasting and the ketogenic diet are high on the list. They are currently the most successful weight loss methods that are relatively easy to integrate into everyday life and ensure weight gains in the long term. The combination of the two is a challenge that requires a new level of discipline. But: It is possible - because: There are two nutritional concepts based on different methods. While keeping your focus on the keto diet on a high-fat and low-carbohydrate diet, interval fasting works on a schedule. Means: For example, you completely do without food and sweetened drinks for 16 hours and only eat for the following eight hours. During this time, however, you should not eat everything, but here the ketogenic diet is used, which relies on healthy fats (read: salmon, avocados, nuts) and largely eliminates carbohydrates from the menu. Both diets are designed to activate ketosis in the body, which will help you lose weight in the long run.

What happens in ketosis?
Ketosis is a metabolic reaction in the body and means that the organism changes its energy production. He usually draws his range of services from glucose, which enters the body through carbohydrate-rich meals. With the ketogenic diet, however, you remove them from your diet and consciously eat 60 to 75 per cent good fats a day. After around 24 to 72 hours, the glucose stores in the body are used up and the body has to look for a new source of energy: this is where the fats are

used. In the so-called hunger metabolism, the body can still use the fat stores for around 50 days and survive - of course; you don't want to bring about this condition, which is why you provide it with an extra dose of fats. So he works with the reserves that we want to get rid of on the abdomen, hips and bottom and reacts in the long term with weight loss. Both the ketogenic diet and interval fasting work with the state of ketosis and want to bring about this other type of metabolism in order to dupe the body - no wonder that a combination of both diets leads to even faster weight loss.

How healthy is this nutritional combination for the body?

While some people's bodies can deal well with ketosis and have few to no side effects, others suffer from lack of sleep, poor concentration, or dry mucous membranes. Especially in the transition phase to the keto diet, some react with flu-like symptoms - here, the body shows how strenuous the new metabolism can be for it. The combination of interval fasting and the ketogenic diet, when used correctly, is not a problem if your own body can handle the available energy and you feel good about it. However, you should discuss the physical constitution with a doctor beforehand in order not to take any health risks. Proper nutrition with lots of fresh food, good fats and fibre also play a role that should not be underestimated. Another difficulty, in the long run, could be that it is difficult to integrate both diets into your everyday life and counteract the weight loss success by increasing exceptions. Therefore, everyone should decide for themselves how realistic the diet combination is for their own lifestyle.

CHAPTER 11
FOODS TO ABSOLUTELY AVOID

Losing weight requires a lot of sacrifice and perseverance, although the most important thing is to follow a healthy diet that allows you to say goodbye to extra pounds. If you want to lose weight, do not lose the detail of the following foods that are totally prohibited and that you should quickly eliminate from your daily diet.

Prohibited foods to lose weight

Sugars

If you are looking to lose some weight, you should not consume any sugar. Sugar is present in foods such as sweets, sugary drinks, jam or fruit juices.

Fats

Saturated fats are totally prohibited in case you are looking to lose a few kilos. That is why you should not consume foods such as sausages, butter or pate.

Fried

Fried foods are other products prohibited in your daily diet. You should avoid batters and products such as croquettes, breaded chicken or fried fish.

Alcohol

Alcohol is a source of calories that contribute nothing and causes the accumulation of fat in the body. That is why you should not drink any alcohol while you want to lose some weight.

Carbs

Foods made from refined flour are totally prohibited if what you want is to lose a few extra pounds of your body.

Ice creams

Although many people believe that they are healthy and perfect foods to drink in the summer, most of them carry a large amount of sugar, which causes enough fat to accumulate in the body. Although it is a product that does not directly fatten, excessive use of salt in meals can cause fluid retention in your body as well as being really harmful to health.

Fruit juices

Most people think that juices are healthy and perfect for the body. The juices have a very large amount of sugar to avoid at all costs if you want to lose a few kilos.

Bread

Bread is a huge source of carbohydrates, so you should moderate your daily consumption. It is advisable to take integral bread since it is much healthier than that made with normal flour.

Dairy Products

Although they also have good properties for the body, dairy products have a high-fat content so they are not advisable in case you want to lose weight. It is much better to opt for skimmed milk products to avoid part of the fat.

Prepared sauces

Ketchup, mustard, barbecues... There are for all tastes, but all of them are characterized by their fatty nature and being highly caloric. If you also take into account a large amount of added sugars, artificial colours, additives and preservatives they contain, it will be better than discarding your daily diet if you want to lose weight. A good alternative is to make the sauces yourself at home with completely natural ingredients. Rich and healthy!

Foods That You Should Include In Your Diet To Lose Weight

Just as there are some foods that you should eliminate from your diet if you are looking for weight loss, there are others that are absolutely recommended to achieve that goal. Take note!

Fruits

In addition to providing a large amount of fibre and being rich in vitamins, fruits help improve digestion and lose abdominal fat. Among them, the following are highly recommended:

- **Apples:** the apple is one of the healthiest fruits that exist.
- **Watermelons:** according to several studies carried out, watermelon lowers body fat and lowers cholesterol.
- **Oranges, lemons, grapefruit, kiwifruit:** the vitamin C present in these fruits makes us process fat faster.
- **Strawberries**: they are not very caloric and also contain a lot of fibre and water.
- **Bananas:** Bananas contain satiating properties which will make you eat less. In addition, they are rich in minerals and quality proteins.

Vegetables

Vegetables should be included in every healthy and balanced diet. Within them, the most beneficial are:

- **Chard, spinach and lettuce:** green vegetables act very effectively against abdominal fat.
- **Celery:** Celery is an excellent food that improves digestion and accelerates metabolism, causing us to lose more calories than we gain. 100% recommended!
- **Tomato:** it is a very low-calorie vegetable very suitable for a balanced diet.

legumes

Some legumes, such as lentils and chickpeas, are ideal for weight loss. They are a source of vegetable protein and help abdominal tone muscles. Of course, it is preferable that you consume them fresh and not canned.

Seafood

Several studies have shown that the monounsaturated fats that seafood contains are perfect for preventing fat accumulation. Still, don't forget to consume it in moderation.

Oatmeal

Highly recommended in diets to lose weight because it contains a high fibre content that absorbs fat and also generates a satiating effect that will make you eat less.

Fish

Fish is rich in vitamins, proteins, minerals and acid grades. To lose weight, enter it in your diet by grilling or baking it.

Golden Rules To Keep In Mind To Lose Weight

The experts are clear: to lose weight and maintain it in the long term; the only key is to follow a varied and balanced diet and accompany it with some physical exercise. Do not forget these premises:

Balance and moderation

The goal of any weight loss plan is to eat fewer calories than the body spends to create a caloric deficit.

Fundamental to do sports

Cardiovascular exercises such as fast walking, cycling or running are the most effective at removing excess fat from the body.

Dieting does not mean starving

The real key is not in quantity but in quality. You should know how to choose well and always opt for those foods that have a low caloric intake.

It's not about dieting, but about changing habits

It is useless for you to spend three months on a demanding and restrictive regimen if afterwards, you will return to the same inadequate diet as always. If what you want, in addition to losing weight, is to maintain it in the long term, you should not understand the diet as a special way of feeding during a specific period, but as a change of habits for a lifetime.

Compensation law applies

If one day you spend on lunch, for example, you can try to eat lighter dinner to compensate and thus not affect the total daily calories.

Don't skip meals

The only thing you will get like this is to arrive with a fierce hunger to the next meal and destroy everything. You will get the opposite effect to the desired one!

Dieting does not mean having to give up meetings with friends and family

In most bars and restaurants, they offer light and healthy alternatives such as salads, vegetable dishes, fish or grilled meats...

Enjoy what you eat

A healthy diet that, at the same time, allows you to lose weight does not have to be boring. Try mixing ingredients, an experiment in the kitchen, create and taste. You will surprise yourself!

CHAPTER 12

INTERMITTENT FASTING RECIPES

LIVER OF HEIFER AND ITS ONION COMPOTE

INGREDIENTS

- 1 slice of organic heifer liver
- 2 small onions
- 1 apple Canada
- tablespoon olive oil
- 1 lemon
- 1 slice of cinnamon
- Salt and pepper

Instruction

1. Peel and slice the onions. Make them return in half of the olive oil until they become translucent. Salt and pepper them. Cover and cook on very low heat for 30 minutes. Watch for cooking, add a little water if necessary.
2. Wash the lemon under running water, wipe it and squeeze it.
3. Wash the apple, peel it, and remove the fibrous core and seeds. Cut it into cubes — Lemon it to avoid blackening place in a

small saucepan with cinnamon and 2 tablespoons water. Cook covered over low heat for 20 minutes. At the end of cooking, crush it in the coarse compote.

4. Cut the liver into strips and cook for 2 to 3 minutes in the pan with the remaining olive oil. Once cooked, mix it with the onion compote.

5. Enjoy it immediately, accompanied by the applesauce.

Nutritional fact

Thanks to the liver, this dish is very rich in iron and zinc, easily assimilated, trace elements essential for the proper functioning of the immune system. It may be particularly recommended for young children, regulated women, and endurance athletes, who often lack iron.

In case of excess cholesterol, do not consume more than one shot per week.

PALETTE OF PORK AND ITS VEGETABLES

INGREDIENTS

- 1 pallet of bone-in pork of 1 kilo
- 100 g smoked diced bacon
- 1/4 green cabbage
- 300 g carrots
- 200 g turnips
- 400 g of firm-fleshed potatoes type BF 15
- 2 onions
- 2 cloves
- 1 bouquet garni
- 1 tablet of organic vegetable broth
- Salt and pepper

Instruction

1. Place the bacon in a saute pan and sauté over medium heat, stirring. Add the palette and use the fat rendered to brown the meat, about 5 minutes on each side. Add a peeled onion and chopped, also brown. Add 1/2 litre of water, the bouquet garni, and the second onion stuck cloves and the crumbled broth.

2. Wash the piece of cabbage, remove the outer leaves too hard, and its core. Dip it in a pan of boiling salted water and let it whiten for 10 minutes. Drain it and cut it

79

into strips. Add it to the sauté pan with the palette, salt, and pepper it, continue cooking for 15 minutes.

3. Wash and peel carrots, turnips, and potatoes. Cut them into slices. Add the carrots and turnips in the pan, salt, and pepper. Continue cooking for 10 minutes. Add the potatoes and finish cooking for 20 minutes. Rectify the seasoning, remove the bouquet garni and onion pique clove.

Nutritional fact

This complete dish simultaneously brings functional meat proteins, fibre, and vitamins from vegetables, energy carbohydrates from potatoes. Low fat, it is suitable for overweight (450 kcal per serving). For a balanced meal, add milk and seasonal fruit.

EXOTIC FRUIT VERRINES

INGREDIENTS

- 2 kiwis
- 1 mango
- 1/2 grenade
- 1/4 litre of semi-skimmed milk
- 2 eggs
- 25 g of sugar
- 1 vanilla pod
- 2 half-sheets of gelatin or 1/2 teaspoon of agar agar

Instruction

1. Wash the vanilla pod, slice it in half, and place it in a saucepan with the milk. Heat and stop the fire just before boiling. Let the vanilla steep in the milk.
2. Position the gelatin in a bowl of cold water.
3. Separate the whites and egg yolks. Whip the yolks with the sugar. Add the cooled and filtered milk. Pour everything into the saucepan and cook on low heat, constantly stirring until the cream thickens. Add drained half-leaves of gelatin or agar-agar, wait for their perfect dissolution to cut the fire. Divide the custard into four glasses and refrigerate for at least 2 hours.

4. Wash the fruits under running water and sponge them out. Peel the kiwis and mango and cut them into cubes. Collect the grains from the pomegranate. Mix these fruits gently and divide them into the glasses. Enjoy it immediately.

Nutritional interest

Thanks to exotic fruits, these verrines are rich in antioxidant vitamins: beta-carotene, vitamins B9, and C, which help the body defend itself against infections.

To balance your menu, consume a verrine at the end of a meal with vegetables, meat, fish or legumes, and starchy foods.

CHICKPEA SALAD

INGREDIENTS

- 150 g chickpeas
- 1 onion
- 1 clove
- 1 clove of garlic
- 1 bouquet garni
- 200 g celery-branch
- 1 lemon
- 5 tablespoons of olive oil
- 1 tip of curry
- 1 tablespoon chopped chives
- Salt and pepper

INSTRUCTION

1. Position the chickpeas in a large bowl filled with cold water and let them soak for 12 hours.
2. Peel the onion and garlic. Drain the chickpeas. Place them in a casserole with 1/2 litre of cold water, the bouquet garni, and the onion stuck clove, the clove of garlic, some grains of pepper. Cover, cook for 2 hours.
3. Wash the celery, detach its branches from the bulb, remove the top of the leaves, detail it in the sticks.

4. Wash the lemon and squeeze its juice — mix 2 tablespoons with the olive oil and the curry.
5. Drain the chickpeas well. Mix with celery. Add salt and pepper. Season with the olive oil vinaigrette and add the chives.

Nutritional fact

This salad, rich in fibre and protein (chickpeas) is very satiating and has a low glycemic index. It can be especially recommended in case of diabetes. Calorie intake reasonable 250 kcal per serving. It is suitable for overweight.

The consumption of pulses is recommended at least twice a week, in order to increase vegetable protein and reduce animal protein.

ROQUEFORT PEAR TOAST

INGREDIENTS

- 8 slices of walnut bread (120 g)
- 1 jar of 100 g of white cheese with 3% fat
- 60 g of Roquefort cheese
- 2 ripe Williams or Guyot pears
- 1 lemon
- 4 nuts

INSTRUCTIONS

1. Toast the slices of bread.
2. Remove the nuts from their shells.
3. Mix together the cottage cheese and Roquefort cheese. Spread toast with this mixture.
4. Wash the lemon, sponge it, and squeeze its juice.
5. Wash the pears, peel them, remove their central part and their pips, divide them into tiny dice. Lemon immediately to prevent the pears from turning black.
6. Spread the pears over the toasts. Add a walnut kernel per toast.

Nutritional fact

Made from walnut bread, Roquefort pear toasts provide 25% of the recommended daily intake of omega 3 essential fats, which are beneficial for cardiovascular prevention. They are rich in fibre (bread, pear, nuts), satiating, and regulating the transit.

Spread with lean fresh cheese with 3% fat and a small amount of Roquefort, they are suitable for hypercholesterolemia.

Whether you eat them as a starter or as an appetizer, you can balance your meal by moderating starchy foods and preparing vegetables.

SHORTBREAD WITH JAM

INGREDIENTS

- 100 g of wheat flour type 55
- 50 g butter or margarine rich in omega 3 not lightened
- 50 g of sugar
- 1 egg
- 120 g of strawberry or apricot jam, homemade if possible
- 2 tablespoons icing sugar
- 1 large star-shaped cookie cutter
- 1 round-shaped cookie cutter 1.5 cm in diameter

INSTRUCTIONS

1. Separate the whites from the egg yolk.
2. In a bowl, mix the flour, sugar, and butter until you have a texture of sand. Add the egg yolk to mix the dough ball. Let the dough rest in the refrigerator for at least 30 minutes.
3. Preheat the oven to 180 ° C. Arrange a sheet of baking paper on a baking sheet.
4. Spread the dough. Cut star-shaped shortbread. In half of these shortbreads, cut a small circle of dough in the middle.

5. Arrange the shortbread on the plate and bake for 15 minutes.
6. Let the shortbread a little cool. Cover each shortbread with jam and sprinkle each shortbread with icing sugar. Arrange the shortbreads pierced over jammed biscuits.

Nutritional fact

Made with flour and jam, these biscuits are rich in carbohydrates and energy. They have their place at the end of a meal without starch or snack after a light lunch. They can also be used as a snack, in recovery after a sports training.

Low in fat, they are suitable for hypercholesterolemia.

SKEWERS OF SEITAN

INGREDIENTS

- 1 block of seitan 240 g
- 1 lemon
- 3 tablespoons sesame oil
- 2 onions
- 1 clove of garlic
- 1 tablespoon acacia honey
- 1 tablespoon paprika
- 200 g cherry tomatoes
- 100 g of Paris mushrooms
- 2 tablespoons sesame seeds
- Salt and pepper

INSTRUCTIONS

1. Wash the lemon under running water, sponge it, and squeeze it.
2. Peel the onions, slice them. Peel and slice the clove of garlic.
3. Cut the seitan into cubes.
4. Mix honey and lemon juice, add oil and paprika, salt, and pepper. Arrange the seitan, onions, and garlic in a dish and sprinkle with the marinade. Allow in the refrigerator for at least 1 hour.
5. Wash the tomatoes and mushrooms, sponge them out. Cut the mushrooms into strips.

6. Make skewers by alternating seitan cubes with onion rings, cherry tomatoes, and mushroom slices. Filter the marinade.

7. Cook the kebabs on a pan in their marinade, 2 min 30 on each side over medium heat. Drain them and roll them in the sesame seeds. Iron for 1 min in the pan, just time to lightly brown the sesame seeds.

Nutritional fact

These skewers provide as much protein as a small steak, the quality of which can be optimized by combining legume proteins, such as lentils. With a reasonable energy intake of 280 kcal, they are suitable for overweight.

BEAN SALAD TO SHELL

INGREDIENTS

- 150 g of shelling beans
- 30 g pasta, farfalle type
- 150 g fresh green beans
- 200 g tomatoes
- 1 carrot
- 1 bouquet garni
- 4 tablespoons olive oil
- 2 tablespoons balsamic vinegar
- 1/2 teaspoon of mustard
- 1 shallot
- 2 teaspoons chopped parsley
- 1 teaspoon chopped basil
- Salt and pepper

INSTRUCTIONS

1. Shell the beans. Position them in a large saucepan and cover them completely with cold water. Add the bouquet garni, cover the pan. Let it simmer for 35 minutes.
2. Wash the green beans and mop them up. Cut in half, salt, and steam for 15 minutes.
3. Cook the pasta the time indicated on the package.
4. Peel and chop the shallot.

5. Prepare the vinaigrette with oil, vinegar, mustard, salt, and pepper. Add the shallot.
6. Wash tomatoes and carrot under running water. Rind off and grate the carrot, cut the tomatoes into wedges.
7. In a salad bowl, combine the shelling beans and the drained pasta, the green beans, the tomatoes, the carrot, and the herbs. Add the vinaigrette and mix gently. Correct the seasoning if necessary.

Nutritional fact

This salad is rich in fibre and antioxidants: vitamin E, vitamin C, lycopene (tomatoes), beta-carotene (carrot). It combines the complementary proteins of beans to shelling and pasta. By doubling the proportions, you will get a balanced vegetarian main course.

RASPBERRY TARTLETS WITHOUT GLUTEN

INGREDIENTS

- 100 g of rice flour
- 30 g of almond powder
- 30 g butter or margarine rich in omega 3 not lightened
- 90 g of sugar
- 2 eggs
- 20 g of cornflower
- 25 cl of semi-skimmed milk
- 1 vanilla pod
- 500 g raspberries
- 1 tablespoon icing sugar

INSTRUCTIONS

1. Heat the milk until boiling. Cut the fire. Split the vanilla pod in half and let it steep in the milk.
2. Mix the rice flour with the almond powder and 60 g sugar. Add the melted butter and work the dough with a fork until you get a sandy texture. Combine the dough with 1 beaten egg and refrigerate for at least 30 minutes.
3. Separate the white and yellow from the remaining egg. Whip the yolk with 30 g of sugar. Add the cornflower, then the milk,

previously filtered, very gradually. Cook this cream over low heat, constantly stirring until thickened (about 3 minutes).

4. Preheat the oven to 180 ° C. Spread the pie dough and divide it into four lightly greased tart pans. Cover each tart with parchment paper and dried vegetables — Cook the tarts for 25 minutes.

5. Wash the raspberries under a stream of running water. Sponge them carefully and remove their peduncles.

6. Wait until the tartlets are cold to garnish with pastry cream and raspberries. Sprinkle with icing sugar.

Nutritional fact

Made from rice flour and corn, this tart is suitable for gluten intolerance. Thanks to raspberries, it is a good source of fibre and vitamin C. Energetic; it has its place at the end of a meal without starchy foods.

QUICHE WITH RATATOUILLE

INGREDIENTS

- 250g of flour
- 125 g butter or margarine rich in omega 3 not lightened
- 2 zucchini
- 1 eggplant
- 3 tomatoes
- 1 yellow pepper
- 1 onion
- 2 tablespoons olive oil
- 1 bouquet garni
- 4 eggs
- 100 g grated Emmental cheese
- Salt and pepper

INSTRUCTIONS

1. In a small salad bowl, mix the flour and butter until you have a texture of sand. Add a little salt water to combine the ball of dough. Let stand in the refrigerator for at least 30 minutes.
2. Peel and slice the onion. Wash the vegetables. Peel the zucchini and cut into slices. Cut the eggplant into cubes. Remove the peduncle, seeds and whitish fibrous parts of pepper, cut into strips.

3. Fry the onion with the olive oil in a frying pan. Add pepper, zucchini, and eggplant, brown while stirring. Add the tomatoes, the bouquet garni, salt, and pepper. Cover; simmer on low heat for 20-30 minutes. At the end of cooking, discover to let evaporate the water of constitution of vegetables.

4. Preheat the oven to 200-210 ° C. Spread the dough and place it in a pie dish. Cover with parchment paper and dried vegetables — Cook for 20 minutes.

5. Mix the well-reduced ratatouille with the eggs and Emmental cheese. Pour this mixture onto the pie shell, free of parchment paper. Finish cooking in the oven for 15 minutes.

Nutritional fact

The ratatouille quiche is a complete balanced dish, which can be supplemented with dairy and fresh fruit.

ZUCCHINI/SHRIMP VERRINES

INGREDIENTS

- 2 zucchini
- 2 shallots
- 2 tablespoons olive oil
- 1/4 teaspoon of curry
- 100 g shelled shrimp
- 1 bunch of chervil
- Salt and pepper

INSTRUCTION

1. Peel and mince the shallots.
2. Wash the zucchini, sponge them, peel them, and cut them in small dice.
3. Place the oil in a pan with the curry. Add the shallots and zucchini to make them come back. Add salt and pepper. Cover, cook for 15-20 minutes over low heat. At the end of cooking, if necessary, evaporate the vegetable water.
4. Divide the zucchini fondue into 4 verrines. Add the shrimp on top and decorate with chervil sprigs.

Nutritional fact

Made from ingredients from the Mediterranean diet, this verrine provides multiple antioxidants (vitamins C and E, beta-carotene, polyphenols, and selenium) to protect the health. Very low fat and low in calories (100 kcal per serving), it is particularly suitable for hypercholesterolemia or overweight.

HOMEMADE SAUERKRAUT

INGREDIENTS

- 1 white cabbage, preferably organic
- 2 teaspoons of salt
- 1 teaspoon juniper berries
- 1 teaspoon of peppercorns
- 6 bay leaves
- 2 glass jars of 1 liter with a screw lid

INSTRUCTION

1. Wash the jars and their lid thoroughly.
2. Put away the outer leaves and the core of the cabbage. Cut it into skinny strips.
3. In each jar, alternate layers of cabbage, each with salt, juniper berries, peppercorns, and bay leaves. Pack well.
4. If there is a bit of room at the top of the jar, add water that has been boiled and chilled. Close the jars without screwing them in completely.
5. Leave the jars at room temperature for 2 days, so that the cabbage can ferment. Then, screw them thoroughly and place them in the refrigerator for 1 month before eating. You can keep them for up to 6 months. Once started, consume them within 48 hours.

Nutritional fact

Preparing homemade sauerkraut helps to consume raw. And so, to enjoy more of its vitamins (C and B9 in particular) and natural lactic ferments at the origin of its obtaining. Some of these ferments reach the colon alive and contribute to the functional diversity of the microbiota (intestinal flora), favorable to health.

Namely: 100 g of sauerkraut provides 100% of the daily need for vitamin K, a contribution that must be taken into account by people on anticoagulant therapy.

HOMEMADE YOGURTS WITH A PRESSURE COOKER

INGREDIENTS

- 90cl of semi-skimmed UHT milk
- 1 jar of plain yogurt with whole commercial milk
- 4 tablespoons of skimmed milk powder
- 1 organic orange
- 1 cooking thermometer

INSTRUCTIONS

1. Wash the orange under running water, sponge it with absorbent paper and recover its zest.
2. Place the milk and orange zest in a saucepan, heat to a boil. Then, turn off the heat and let the zest infuse until the milk temperature drops to 45 ° C (check with the thermometer).
3. During this time, fill the pressure cooker with water for one third. Close the lid and put it on the fire. Leave several minutes under pressure. Then, cut the fire and let the steam escape.
4. Sift the milk through the sieve to remove the orange zest. Whisk it with yogurt and milk powder. Divide into 8 glass yogurt jars.

5. Discard the boiling water from the pressure cooker. Place the pots in the basket of the casserole and enclose them immediately in the still very hot casserole. Let it ferment at room temperature for 4 - 5 hours. Then place the yogurt in the refrigerator.

Nutritional fact

Yogurt makes it possible to take advantage of the good proteins and the calcium of the milk, even in case of intolerance to lactose (sugar of cow, goat, and sheep milk), that its lactic ferments have the capacity to digest. It can be called probiotic, because its regular consumption contributes to the development, within the microbiota (intestinal flora), of bacteria considered as beneficial to health.

OMELET WITH CHICKEN LIVERS

INGREDIENTS

- 6 eggs
- 150 g of chicken livers
- 2 shallots
- 3 tablespoons of olive oil
- 1 tsp chopped parsley, 1 teaspoon chopped chives, 1 tsp chopped tarragon
- Salt and pepper

INSTRUCTIONS

1. Pare and cut in 4 the chicken livers. Peel and mince the shallots.
2. Fry the chicken livers in the olive oil and cook for 3 to 4 minutes. Then, reserve them and sweat the shallots over a fairly soft fire. Mix them with the livers and reserve.
3. Beat the eggs, salt and pepper them. Cook them in a sloppy omelet. Spread over the chicken livers and herbs.
4. Fold the omelet and slide it onto a serving dish.

Nutritional fact

Poultry liver omelet provides good protein that is effective for growing children, as well as maintaining muscle mass in adults. It is a good source of vitamin D: 2g per serving, or 40% of the recommended daily intake.

Its reasonable caloric intake (225 kcal) allows us to consume it in case of overweight.

To know: this recipe is not recommended for pregnant women and children under 3 years because of the very high vitamin A content of chicken livers.

CHEESECAKE

INGREDIENTS

- 350 g of 3% fat (3% fat) white cheese enriched with vitamin D (Calin + type)
- 2 eggs
- 35 g of Maïzena
- 60 g of sugar
- 1 teaspoon of bitter almond extract
- 1 tablespoon flaked almonds
- Salt

INSTRUCTIONS

1. Preheat the oven to 170 ° C. Garnish a mold to run out of baking paper.
2. Separate the yolks and whites from the eggs. Climb these in very firm snow with a pinch of salt.
3. Mix the Maïzena gradually with the cottage cheese. Then add the egg yolks, the sugar, then the almond extract. When the preparation is homogeneous, gently add the egg whites.
4. Pour the dough into the mold and bake for 40 to 45 minutes. Check the cooking by pricking the cake with a knife tip. Wait until it has cooled down to remove the baking paper.

5. Pass the almonds quickly in a non-stick frying pan for browning. Decorate the cake.

Nutritional fact

The cottage cheesecake provides good protein (cottage cheese, egg), as well as energy carbohydrates (sugar, Maizena). Made from white cheese enriched with calcium and vitamin D, it provides respectively 25 and 100% of the recommended daily intake to an adult in these micronutrients. It may be particularly recommended for growing teenagers and seniors for the prevention of osteoporosis.

PEAR AND WALNUT

INGREDIENTS

- 1 beautiful pear
- 80 g of butter
- 1/2 teaspoon of vanilla extract
- 2 eggs
- 100 g of sugar
- 50 g of chestnut flour
- 50 g of wheat flour type 55
- 1/2 sachet of yeast
- 80 g unsweetened cocoa powder
- 14 nuts
- 2 teaspoons icing sugar

INSTRUCTIONS

1. Preheat the oven to 180 - 200 ° C. Lightly grease a non-stick mold with an oiled brush.
2. Wash the pear, peel it, remove its central part and its seeds, cut it in big quarters. Put it in the pan with 20 g of butter and vanilla. Remove it from the fire as soon as it begins to caramelize. Arrange it at the bottom of the mold.
3. Schell nuts.
4. Separate the whites from the egg yolks. Beat the egg whites with a pinch of salt.

5. Mix the egg yolks with the sugar. Add the remaining 60 g of butter. Gradually add the two flours with the yeast, then the cocoa powder, and finally 12 nuts. Carefully incorporate the whites into the snow.

6. Pour the mix into the pan over the pear and bake for 25 minutes at 180 ° C. Check the cooking with a knife tip (the dough does not stick when the cake is cooked).

7. Unmount the pound. Sprinkle with icing sugar and decorate with the remaining 2 nuts.

POTATO SALAD WITH SMOKED HERRING

INGREDIENTS

- 400 g of firm-fleshed potatoes such as Amandine or Belle de Fontenay
- 1 small beet
- 2 shallots
- 150 g sweet smoked herring fillets
- 4 tablespoons ISIO 4 mixed oil
- 2 tablespoons vinegar
- 1 teaspoon of mustard
- 2 teaspoons chopped dill (fresh or frozen)
- Salt and pepper

INSTRUCTIONS

1. Wash the potatoes under running water, peel them, slice them and steam them for 20 minutes.
2. Cut the herring into cubes.
3. Peel the beetroot and cut into cubes. Peel and slice the shallots
4. Mix mustard, oil, vinegar, and shallots.
5. Divide the still-warm potatoes and beet into 4 serving plates: salt very lightly and pepper. Add herring and vinaigrette, sprinkle with dill. Taste immediately.

Nutritional fact

This salad is rich in protein (herring), as well as in fiber and complex carbohydrates (potato). But, his main interests are his contributions of essential omega 3 and vitamin D, abundant in oil ISIO 4 and herring. One serving provides about 12 grams of vitamin D, more than double the recommended daily intake.

This salad is suitable for diabetes or overweight (250 kcal per person), provided it is consumed within a balanced meal, combined with a good vegetable dish, a dairy, and fresh seasonal fruit.

SALMON WITH LENTILS

INGREDIENTS

- 1 salmon steak
- 50 g du Puy lentils
- 1 carrot
- 1 onion
- 1 bouquet garni
- 1 small white leek
- 1 teaspoon dried tomatoes
- 1 shallot
- 1 tablespoon olive oil
- 1 tablespoon dry white wine
- Salt and pepper

INSTRUCTIONS

1. Wash the carrot and peel it. Peel the onion. Cut these vegetables into large slices. Place them with the lentils and the bouquet garni in a saucepan. Cover with cold water, cover, and cook for 30 minutes in small broths. Salt at the end of cooking and remove bouquet garni and slices of vegetables.

2. Wash the leek and thinly slice it. Peel and chop the shallot. Sweat these vegetables with olive oil. Then add the white wine and 2 tablespoons water, cover, cook on low heat for 20 minutes. Add the dried

tomatoes, a little water if necessary, and finish cooking 10 min.
3. Steam the salmon for 10 minutes.
4. Arrange salmon and lentils on a serving platter. Spread over the leek fondue.

Nutritional fact

Very rich in proteins (salmon, lentils) and fiber (lentils, vegetables), this main course is particularly satisfying. Associated with a dairy and a fruit, it allows us to "hold" without hunger until the next meal and so not to nibble. It is particularly suitable for diabetes or overweight (510 kcal per serving).

SPINACH EGG CAKE

INGREDIENTS

- 1 commercial buckwheat pancake
- 150 g spinach
- 1 egg
- 1 tablespoon of olive oil
- 1 teaspoon chopped parsley
- Salt and pepper

INSTRUCTIONS

1. Wash the spinach under running water with a strainer. Drain them in a dishcloth or salad spinner. Remove their tail and ribs if necessary. Place in a pan with olive oil, salt, and pepper. Let them cook for 5 minutes on high heat, just until their water evaporates. Reserve them.

2. Place the pancake in the pan so that it warms up. Garnish with spinach. Break the egg over the center, salt, and pepper. As soon as the white is cooked, remove the pan from the heat.

3. Sprinkle with parsley and fold the 4 corners of the cake. Enjoy it immediately.

Nutritional fact

The egg whip spinach is a complete dish, which simultaneously provides good protein (egg), energy complex carbohydrates (buckwheat), and vegetables. Thanks to spinach, it is particularly rich in beta-carotene (100% of the recommended daily intake of an adult), vitamins C and B9 (50% of the recommended intake). It also provides a quarter of the daily needs of fiber and calcium.

Not very fat, it has a reasonable energy intake: 290 kcal, it is suitable for overweight.

In cases of high cholesterol, remember to count the egg in your weekly quota.

CUPS OF STRAWBERRIES WITH MANGO

INGREDIENTS

- 400 g strawberries
- 1 mango
- 60 g frozen blackcurrant kernels
- 2 teaspoons honey all flowers
- 4 tablespoons of homemade pressed orange juice or fresh ray
- 1 tablespoon of silver-colored sugar pearls
- 4 lace pancakes

INSTRUCTIONS

1. A few hours in advance, place the black currants in the refrigerator to thaw.
2. Wash the strawberries under running water, pat them well with paper towels and shake them off. Wash the mango under running water and sponge it.
3. Mix the honey with the orange juice.
4. Cut the mango in half (cut flush with the core). Peel each half and cut into cubes. Cut the strawberries in half. Delicately mix mango, strawberries, blackcurrant, and orange sauce. Divide the fruit salad into 4 cups. Garnish with sugar pearls and arrange a lace crepe in each cup. Enjoy it immediately.

Nutritional fact

The strawberry mango cut combines 4 fruits richest in vitamin C so that a serving represents 80% of the recommended daily intake to an adult. It is also a healthy source of beta-carotene (especially thanks to mango), vitamin B9, and fiber: 15% of the recommended intake for each of these nutrients.

Providing potassium and simple sugars, based on fruits with alkalizing virtues, it can be offered in recovery after an effort to children or adult athletes.

COCONUT-PINEAPPLE MOUSSE

INGREDIENTS

- 3 eggs
- 37.5 cl of coconut milk
- 60 g of sugar
- 1/4 to 1/3 pineapple (200 g net)
- 5 half-sheets of gelatin
- 1 pinch of salt

INSTRUCTIONS

1. Separate the yolks and egg whites.
2. Soak the gelatin in a bowl of cold water.
3. Whip the egg yolks with the sugar. Gradually add the coconut milk. Put everything into a saucepan and cook on low heat, constantly stirring until the cream is tableclothed.
4. Drain the gelatin carefully and add it to the coconut cream. Whip, and as soon as the gelatin is dissolved, remove the pan from the heat. Let cool for 1 hour in the refrigerator.
5. Peel the pineapple: remove its skin. It's the central hard part and its "eyes." Make sure you have 200 g of flesh that you cut into small cubes.

117

6. Add a pinch of salt to the egg whites and beat in the snow firmly. Mix them gently with the coconut cream. Add the pineapple dice. Divide the mousse into 4 ramekins and put in at least 2 hours in the refrigerator before eating.

Nutritional fact

Thanks to coconut milk, the coconut-pineapple mousse is rich in potassium, vegetable iron, and vitamin B5. Thanks to the eggs, it provides proteins of excellent nutritional quality. Coconut milk is good and high in saturated fat (17%), but it is mainly lauric acid, which, according to recent studies, does not affect the blood cholesterol level.

SPINACH GRATIN WITH GOAT CHEESE

INGREDIENTS

- 250 g fresh spinach
- 1 teaspoon of butter (10 g)
- 1 teaspoon flour (10 g)
- 10 cl of goat's milk
- 30 g fresh goat cheese
- Nutmeg
- Salt and pepper

INSTRUCTION

1. Wash the spinach under running water, sponge them out, mop them up. Place them in a pan with salt and pepper, cover, cook on low heat for 15 minutes.
2. Preheat the oven to 200 ° C.
3. Place the butter and sifted the flour in a saucepan. Mix over low heat. Add the milk gradually. Salt and pepper, grate some nutmeg. Cook over low heat, constantly stirring for some minutes.
4. Mix the bechamel with the well-drained spinach. Arrange everything in an individual gratin dish Emit the goat cheese over it — Bake in the oven for about some minutes.

Nutritional fact

Thanks to spinach, this gratin is rich in vegetable iron, vitamins E and K, anti-oxidant carotenoids, and fiber. Enriched with milk and goat cheese, it provides nearly 400 mg of calcium or 45% of the recommended daily intake to an adult. This dish is particularly suitable for children, teenagers, pregnant women (if you choose a cheese made from pasteurized milk), and the elderly.

EGGS WITH MILK AND GOAT CHEESE

INGREDIENTS

- 2 eggs
- 40 cl whole goat's milk
- 60 g Pouligny-Saint-Pierre (goat cheese)
- 2 slices of Bayonne ham (60 g)
- Pepper

INSTRUCTIONS

1. Preheat the oven to 180 ° C.
2. Cut the cheese into small cubes. Slice the ham in chiffonade.
3. Beat the eggs in an omelet. Add the milk gradually. Add the diced goat cheese, ham, and a little pepper.
4. Divide the resulting preparation into four individual ramekins. Arrange the ramekins in an oven dish in which you have poured the bottom of the water so that the milk eggs cook in a bain-marie.
5. Bake for 30 minutes at 180 ° C. Check the cooking of the eggs with a knife tip (the preparation does not stick when the eggs are cooked).

Nutritional fact

Milk and goat eggs are rich in high-quality protein for growth as well as muscle maintenance. Can be served as a main dish, replacing the meat.

Thanks to milk and goat cheese, they provide vitamins B2, B12, A, and D, as well as calcium: 150 mg per serving, or 17% of the recommended daily intake.

They are especially suitable for children, teens, athletes, and the elderly.

PALETS WITH SQUASH SEEDS

INGREDIENTS

- 80 g flour type 55 or 80
- 5 tablespoons of olive oil
- 1/2 teaspoon of baking soda (yeast)
- 40 g squash seeds
- 30 g dried tomatoes
- 1 teaspoon dried oregano
- Salt

INSTRUCTIONS

1. Mix the flour, baking soda, squash seeds, sun-dried tomatoes, and oregano. Include 4 tablespoons of olive oil and 1 pinch of salt. Add a few spoons of water to form a ball of dough. Let stand at least 30 minutes at room temperature.
2. Preheat the oven to 180 ° C. Arrange a sheet of baking paper on a baking sheet. Brush with the remaining oil.
3. Sprinkle with flour the work plan. Roll out the dough as finely as possible with a rolling pin. Use a cookie cutter to cut pucks. Arrange the pucks on the parchment paper. Bake for 15 minutes at 185 ° C. Check the cooking with a knife tip (the dough does not stick when the puck is cooked).

123

Nutritional fact

The squash seeds combine healthy ingredients, useful in cardiovascular prevention: olive oil and squash seeds, high in unsaturated fats that help reduce the level of bad blood cholesterol and tomatoes, including lycopene (which colors them in red) is a powerful antioxidant.

In case of diabetes, know that a portion of these pucks corresponds to 30 g of bread.

WHITING BREAD WITH SESAME

INGREDIENT

- 400 g whiting fillets
- 4 tablespoons sesame oil
- 1 lemon
- 1 tablespoon soy sauce
- 1 clove of garlic
- 2 tablespoons minced lemongrass
- 1 small piece of ginger 1 cm
- 4 tablespoons sesame seeds
- 2 eggs
- Salt and pepper

INSTRUCTIONS

1. Wash the lemon under running water, sponge it, squeeze it. Peel and slice the clove of garlic. Pass the ginger under the water, sponge it, grate it.
2. Prepare a marinade with 2 tablespoons of sesame oil, lemon juice, soy sauce, lemongrass, garlic, ginger, and a little pepper. Arrange the whiting fillets in the marinade and reserve them in the refrigerator for 2 hours.
3. Then very carefully drain the fish fillets. Cook them for 5 minutes, steaming.

4. Separate the egg whites from the yolks. Spread each fillet of whiting in the egg yolk and then in the sesame seeds to form a breadcrumb. Salt slightly. Quickly pass the breaded fish fillets in a non-stick frying pan with the remaining 2 spoons of oil. As soon as the sesame seeds are golden brown, stop cooking. Enjoy it immediately.

Nutritional fact

Whiting is rich in protein of excellent quality for growth, as is the maintenance of muscle mass. Breaded with sesame, it is also an excellent source of calcium, magnesium, and iron. It is suitable for hypercholesterolemia since sesame provides mainly unsaturated fats.

ALMOND/PEAR EXPRESS CREAM

INGREDIENTS

- 1 pot of semi-skimmed milk cheese with 3% fat
- 1 teaspoon of almond powder
- 1/2 teaspoon of flax seeds
- 2 drops of bitter almond extract
- 1 teaspoon of honey
- 1 lemon
- 1 pear
- 1 small square of dark chocolate

INSTRUCTIONS

1. Place the flax seeds in a non-stick pan. Roast them for 2 minutes over medium heat, stirring them, so they do not burn.
2. Wash the lemon under running water, sponge it, and squeeze it.
3. Mix the white cheese with almond powder, bitter almond extract, 2 teaspoons lemon juice, honey, and flax seeds.
4. Wash the pear, peel it, dice it, and lemon it. Mix with almond cream.
5. Slice the chocolate into thin chips and sprinkle the cream. Enjoy it immediately.

Nutritional fact

The almond/pear cream is a good source of calcium, particularly recommended for growing young people or seniors in the prevention of osteoporosis. Rich in fiber, it is satisfying and useful to regularise the transit. Thanks to flaxseed, it provides 50% of the recommended daily intake of essential Omega 3. As almonds mainly provide monounsaturated fats (the same as in olive oil), it can be supported in cases of hypercholesterolemia.

SEASONAL VEGETABLE CAKE

INGREDIENTS

- 100 g of flour type 55
- 2 eggs
- 3 tablespoons of olive oil
- 300 g of already cooked vegetables: carrots, cauliflower, zucchini, broccoli, spinach, peas ...
- 80 ml of semi-skimmed milk
- 1/2 sachet of yeast
- 40 g of goat cheese
- 40 g of Emmentaler
- 1 teaspoon chopped parsley
- 1 teaspoon chopped mint
- Salt and pepper

INSTRUCTIONS

1. Heat the oven to 200 ° C. Line a small cake tin with parchment paper.
2. Quickly pass the vegetables in the pan with 1 spoon of oil to lightly grill. Season them with the herbs.
3. Mix the flour with the yeast, then the eggs. Gradually add the milk and the remaining 2 spoons of oil. Add salt and pepper. Finish by incorporating vegetables, diced goat cheese, and grated Emmental cheese.

4. Pour the mix into the cake pan and bake for 30 minutes. Check the cooking with a knife tip (when the cake is cooked, the dough does not stick to the knife).

Nutritional fact

The seasonal vegetable cake is an energy starter rich in complex carbohydrates and protein.

In case of diabetes, one serving replaces 40 g of bread (1/6 of baguette) or 100 g of starch (3 tablespoons). In the case of hypercholesterolemia, avoid consuming other cheese during the day.

ZUCCHINI FLAN

INGREDIENTS

- 1 zucchini
- 1 tomato
- 1 shallot
- 1 teaspoon of olive oil
- 1 pinch of oregano
- 1 egg
- 2 tablespoons cottage cheese
- 1 tablespoon thick cream
- 1 teaspoon Maïzena
- 1 tablespoon grated Emmental cheese
- Salt and pepper

INSTRUCTIONS

1. Wash the zucchini and tomato under running water, pat them and peel them. Remove the fibrous central part of the tomato and cut it into quarters. Cut the zucchini into thin slices.

2. Peel and chop the shallot. Sweat over fairly low heat in olive oil for a few minutes, then add the zucchini and tomato. Add salt, pepper, and oregano, cover and cook for 15 minutes on low heat. At the end of cooking, discover the vegetables to reduce them well.

131

3. Preheat the oven to 180 ° C. Beat the omelet egg and mix it with the Fromage blanc, the cream, and the Maïzena. Add salt and pepper.
4. Place the vegetables in the bottom of an individual gratin dish. Cover them with gratin and sprinkle with grated cheese — Bake for 15 minutes at 180 ° C.

Nutritional fact

The zucchini custard is a complete dish, which can be combined with a slice of bread and fruit for a balanced meal.

It helps to provide good protein (egg, cottage cheese, Emmental) to those who have difficulty in eating meat, including the elderly.

MUSHROOM CAKE AO-NORI

INGREDIENTS

- 80 g of buckwheat flour
- 5 eggs
- 600 g mushrooms from Paris
- 2 shallots
- 2 cloves garlic
- 2 tablespoons olive oil
- 40 g of ao-nori (green algae) in the jar
- 1 tablespoon chopped parsley
- 1 tablespoon of sunflower oil
- Salt and pepper

INSTRUCTIONS

1. Prepare the dough by mixing the buckwheat flour with 20 cl of water, a nice pinch of salt, and 1/4 egg beaten into an omelet. Cover the salad bowl and let the dough rest in the refrigerator for 1 hour.

2. Drain and slice the ao-nori. Peel and slice garlic and shallots. Wash the mushrooms under running water, remove their earthy foot, cut them into slices. In a pan, sauté garlic, shallots, and mushrooms with olive oil. Salt and pepper, sprinkle with ao-nori. Cook for 10 minutes (all the mushrooms

    water must be evaporated) and add the parsley.

3. Bake 4 patties in a lightly greased non-stick pan with an oiled brush.

4. Spread the pan-fried mushrooms on 4 patties. Iron each pancake in the pan. Break an egg in the center. Once the white is cooked, fold the edges of the cake to give it a square shape and serve it immediately.

Nutritional fact

The mushroom cake ao-nori is a complete dish: it provides complex energy carbohydrates (flour), proteins (eggs), and fiber (mushrooms, algae). Thanks to the ao-nori, it is a good source of iron and iodine.

Its energy intake is reasonable: 280 kcal per galette. It can be consumed in case of the celiac disease since buckwheat does not contain gluten.

VEGETABLE TOAST

INGREDIENTS

- 30 g chickpeas
- 1 big tomato "Heart of beef" (200 to 250 g)
- 30 g red pepper
- 1 clove of garlic
- 1 teaspoon chopped parsley
- 3 teaspoons of olive oil
- 1/2 teaspoon chopped basil
- 1 nice slice of country bread (50 to 60 g)
- Salt and pepper

INSTRUCTIONS

1. Soak the chickpeas in cold water for an hour. The next day, drain them carefully and allow them to dry thoroughly before cooking.
2. Peel the garlic. Wash the piece of pepper, remove its whitish fibrous parts and seeds. Wash the tomato, remove the fibrous central part.
3. Mix together the chickpeas, the clove of garlic, the piece of pepper, 50 g of tomato, the parsley, salt, and pepper. Shape the slab-shaped dough the size of the minced steak and pan fry with 2 tablespoons olive oil 3 minutes on each side.

4. Grill the slice of country bread.
5. Cut the remaining tomato into carpaccio.
6. Arrange half of the tomato carpaccio on the slice of bread, drizzle with olive oil, season with salt, pepper, and basil. Put over the chickpea galette. Finish with the rest of the carpaccio season. Enjoy it immediately.

Nutritional fact

Vegetable bread is a complete balanced dish. It is rich in protein, energy complex carbohydrates (bread, chickpeas), fiber, vitamin C, and anti-oxidant lycopene (tomato). It combines many ingredients of the Mediterranean diet, protectors of the cardiovascular system.

PEACH FONDANT

INGREDIENTS

- 2 pears Conference
- 2 eggs
- 1/4 liter of semi-skimmed milk
- 2 tablespoons maple syrup or 3 teaspoons of sugar
- 1 lemon
- 30 g oat flakes
- 1 vanilla pod
- 2 tablespoons rum
- 2 level tablespoons of flaked almonds

INSTRUCTIONS

1. Spread the vanilla pod under the water, then slice it in half and place it with the milk in a saucepan. Heat to a boil, then turn off the heat and let the vanilla brew.
2. Preheat the oven to 180 ° C.
3. Mix the oatmeal. Remove the vanilla pod from cooled milk and gradually mix milk and oatmeal. Add the maple syrup, the rum, then the 2 beaten egg omelet.
4. Wash the lemon and squeeze it. Wash the pears, cut them in half, remove the fibrous central part and the pips, peel them. Lemon them immediately to avoid blackening them.

Arrange the 4 half-pears in a gratin dish. Pour over the milk mixture.

5. Bake for 30 minutes at 180 ° C. Check the cooking with a knife tip.

6. Quickly brown the flaked almonds in a non-stick frying pan and decorate the fondant.

Nutritional fact

Not very sweet, high in fiber with pears and oatmeal, this low-glycemic dessert is suitable for diabetes. Providing only 190 kcal per serving, it can also be consumed in case of overweight.

EXOTIC FRUIT VERRINES

INGREDIENTS

- 2 kiwis
- 1 mango
- 1/2 grenade
- 1/4 liter of semi-skimmed milk
- 2 eggs
- 25 g of sugar
- 1 vanilla pod
- 2 half-sheets of gelatin or 1/2 teaspoon of agar agar

INSTRUCTIONS

1. Wash the vanilla pod, slice it in half, and place it in a saucepan with the milk. Heat and stop the fire just before boiling. Let the vanilla steep in the milk.
2. Position the gelatin in a bowl of cold water.
3. Separate the whites and egg yolks. Whip the yolks with the sugar. Add the cooled and filtered milk. Pour everything into the saucepan and cook on low heat, continually stirring until the cream thickens. Add drained half-leaves of gelatin or agar-agar, wait for their complete dissolution to cut the fire. Divide the custard into four glasses and refrigerate for at least 2 hours.

4. Wash the fruits under running water and sponge them out. Peel the kiwis and mango and cut them into cubes. Collect the grains from the pomegranate. Mix these fruits gently and divide them into the glasses. Enjoy it immediately.

SHORTBREAD WITH JAM

INGREDIENTS

- 100 g of wheat flour type 55
- 50 g butter or margarine rich in omega 3 not lightened
- 50 g of sugar
- 1 egg
- 120 g of strawberry or apricot jam, homemade if possible
- 2 tablespoons icing sugar
- 1 large star-shaped cookie cutter
- 1 round-shaped cookie cutter 1.5 cm in diameter

INSTRUCTIONS

1. Separate the whites from the egg yolk.
2. In a bowl, mix the flour, sugar, and butter until you have a texture of sand. Add the egg yolk to mix the dough ball. Let the dough rest in the refrigerator for at least 30 minutes.
3. Preheat the oven to 180 ° C. Arrange a sheet of baking paper on a baking sheet.
4. Spread the dough. Cut star-shaped shortbread. In half of these shortbreads, cut a small circle of dough in the middle.

5. Arrange the shortbread on the plate and bake for 15 minutes.
6. Let the shortbread a little cool. Cover each shortbread with jam and sprinkle each shortbread with icing sugar. Arrange the shortbreads pierced over jammed biscuits.

Nutritional fact

Made with flour and jam, these biscuits are rich in carbohydrates and energy. They have their place at the end of a meal without starch or snack after a light lunch. They can also be used as a snack, in recovery after a sports training.

Low in fat, they are suitable for hypercholesterolemia.

CHOCOLATE PEAR CHARLOTTE

INGREDIENTS

- 18 biscuits with a spoon
- 1 tablespoon liquid vanilla extract
- 2 beautiful ripe pears
- 2 jars of chocolate cream-dessert (250 g)
- 1 lemon
- 1 tablespoon chocolate granules

INSTRUCTIONS

1. Wash the lemon under running water, sponge it, and squeeze it.
2. Wash the pears, peel them, and remove any excessively ripe parts. Cut them into cubes. Place them in a small saucepan with the lemon juice. Cook them covered over low heat for 20 minutes. At the end of cooking, crush them in the sauce.
3. Mix the vanilla extract with 4 tablespoons of water. Dip the biscuits very quickly in the vanilla and line the bottom and edges of 4 ramekins. Spread half of the cooled compote on the biscuits. Pour over the chocolate cream (a 1/2 pot per ramekin). Finish with the remaining compote. Place the charlottes in the refrigerator for at least 4 hours.

143

4. Unmould the charlottes just before serving and decorate them with chocolate granules.

Nutritional fact

The charlotte pear/chocolate is a dessert or energetic snack rich in carbohydrates. Thanks the pears, it has good fiber and potassium content.

Very low fat, it is suitable for hypercholesterolemia.

It provides 250 kcal per serving: if you watch your line, take it at the end of a meal without starch.

POACHED APRICOTS WITH BLACKCURRANT

INGREDIENTS

- 2 apricots
- 10 cl of pure blackcurrant juice
- 1 slice of gingerbread
- 1/2 vanilla pod
- 2 teaspoons of aspartame or sucralose powder

INSTRUCTIONS

1. Rinse the vanilla bean under running water and cut in half.
2. Place the blackcurrant juice and vanilla in a small saucepan. Heat until the first tremors, then let the vanilla brew at least 30 minutes.
3. Wash the apricots, pit them, and separate the mumps. Place them in the blackcurrant juice and let them cook for 15 minutes over low heat.
4. At the end of cooking, add the sweetener, remove the vanilla, and then discover the pan so that the blackcurrant juice is reduced.
5. Arrange the slice of gingerbread on a dessert plate. Add the apricot mumps. Sprinkle with blackcurrant syrup.
6. Allow cooling well before eating.

Nutritional fact

Based on apricots and cassis, this dessert is rich in anti-oxidants: beta-carotene (pro-vitamin A) and anthocyanins (dark red pigments) that act synergistically in the body. "Sweet" with a sweetener, it has a reasonable energy intake: 145 kcal per serving.

For a balanced meal, precede your poached apricots with meat, fish, and vegetables (or mixed salad) and dairy.

BAVARIAN VANILLA/COFFEE

INGREDIENTS

- 1/2 liter of semi-skimmed milk
- 4 egg yolks
- 3 tablespoons of aspartame-based sweetener or sucralose
- 1 vanilla pod
- 2 teaspoons instant coffee
- 4 half -sheets of gelatin
- 1 tablespoon flaked almonds

INSTRUCTIONS

1. Soak 2 half-sheets of gelatin in a bowl of cold water.
2. Heat 1/4 liter of milk with the vanilla pod. When boiling, remove the milk from the heat and let the vanilla brew while it cools.
3. Separate the whites and yolks from 2 eggs.
4. Whisk the yolks, place them in a saucepan and add the cooled milk very gradually. Cook this mixture on low heat, constantly stirring, until the cream coats the spoon. Remove the vanilla bean and add half of the sweetener and the drained gelatin. Whip until the perfect dissolution of the gelatin.
5. Divide the vanilla cream into 4 ramekins and refrigerate for 2 hours.

6. Prepare another coffee cream which you will pour gently into the ramekins and take 2 hours again.
7. Just before serving, quickly pass the almonds in a nonstick skillet for browning and decorating the bavarois.

Nutritional fact

Bavarian is rich in calcium (milk) and protein (milk, egg). Based on semi-skimmed milk and sweetener, its calorie intake is reasonable: 115 kcal per serving. Without sugar, it is suitable for people with diabetes. In case of high cholesterol, consider counting the yolk among your eggs of the week.

CLAFOUTIS MULTI FRUITS

INGREDIENTS

- 400 g (net) of seasonal fruits: peaches, apricots, cherries
- 20 cl of semi-skimmed milk
- 2 eggs
- 40 g flour (2 tablespoons)
- 40 g sugar (2 tablespoons)
- 1 teaspoon liquid vanilla extract

INSTRUCTIONS

1. Wash the fruits under running water. Stake and pit the cherries. Peel the peaches. If the fruit is very ripe, remove any damaged parts. Cut them into small cubes.
2. Preheat the oven to 180 ° C.
3. Beat the omelet eggs and add the sugar. Then gradually add the sifted flour. Finish with milk and vanilla extract.
4. Mix the clafoutis with the fruits. Pour the mixture into an oven pan. Bake for 180 ° C for 30 minutes: check the cooking with a knife tip or a baking needle (the clafoutis is cooked when its dough does not stick to the tip of the knife).

Nutritional fact

Clafoutis multi fruits can take advantage of the good fruit nutrients (except vitamin C degraded by heat): fiber, potassium, beta-carotene, and antioxidant polyphenols. Thanks to eggs and milk, it provides good quality protein and calcium. It is an interesting dessert for children or teenagers who have difficulty eating fruit at the table.

Its energy intake is reasonable: 225 kcal the portion.

LEEK GRATIN

INGREDIENTS

- 2 leeks
- 1 teaspoon of butter
- 1 teaspoon Maïzena
- 12 cl of whole milk
- 50 g grated Emmental cheese
- Nutmeg
- Salt and pepper

INSTRUCTIONS

1. Wash the leeks carefully; remove their earthy foot and their green. Cut the whites into pieces and place them in a steamer. Salt them and cook for 25 minutes. Once cooked, let them drain well.
2. Preheat the grill in the oven.
3. Mix the butter and Maïzena. Place them over low heat in a small saucepan to obtain a white roux. Add the milk with a whisk.
4. Add grated nutmeg and half of the Emmental cheese at the end of cooking. Salt lightly and pepper.
5. Arrange the leeks in the bottom of an individual gratin dish. Cover with Mornay sauce and sprinkle with remaining Emmental cheese.

151

Nutritional fact

- Thanks to milk and Emmental, leek gratin is very rich in calcium: (600 mg per serving, or 50% of the recommended intake for over 50s) and protein of excellent quality.
- Thanks to leeks, it also provides fiber, potassium, and carotenoids with antioxidant properties.
- This dish is particularly adapted to the needs of teenagers, pregnant women, and seniors.

GLUTEN-FREE CHOCOLATE FONDANT

INGREDIENTS

- 100 g of dark chocolate pastry
- 50 g of butter
- 50 g of sugar
- 1 egg
- 40 g of Maïzena
- 1 teaspoon of natural vanilla extract
- 4 individual non-stick molds

INSTRUCTIONS

1. Heat the oven to 180 ° C.
2. Separate the whites from the egg yolk. Add a pinch of salt to the whites and beat in the snow.
3. Cut the chocolate into squares and butter into cubes. Place these two ingredients in a large bowl and microwave in the oven for 1 minute to melt. Mix them well with a whisk.
4. Mix the egg yolk with the sugar. Add the sifted Maïzena, beat well. Then add the chocolate and butter mixture, as well as the vanilla extract. Finally, gently add the white to snow.
5. Divide the dough into the 4 molds — Bake for 10 minutes at 180 ° C.

LIGHT TOMATO PIE

INGREDIENTS

- 4 sheets of brick
- 600 g tomatoes
- 1 beautiful onion
- 1 clove of garlic
- 3 tablespoons of olive oil
- 2 tablespoons of a dry white wine
- 1 bouquet garni
- 1 teaspoon of Provence herbs
- 4 eggs
- 1 mozzarella ball
- Salt and pepper

INSTRUCTIONS

1. Peel and slice garlic and onion. Wash the tomatoes under running water, peel them, remove the fibrous core and cut them into wedges.
2. Fry garlic, onion, and tomatoes in 2 tablespoons olive oil. Add the white wine, the bouquet garni, the herbs of Provence, salt, and pepper. Cover, simmer on low heat for 20 minutes. Add some water during cooking if necessary and let reduce at the end of cooking. Take off the bouquet garni.
3. Preheat the thermostat oven 6/7 (200 ° C).

4. Position a sheet of parchment paper in the bottom of a pie plate for four people. Cover with a sheet of brick that you brush with olive oil with a brush. Arrange the other three sheets of brick in the same way.
5. Mix the tomato coulis with the beaten egg omelet. Correct the seasoning if necessary. Arrange this device on the filo paste. Finish with the sliced mozzarella. Bake 15 minutes.

Nutritional fact

The light tomato pie is a complete dish, providing proteins (eggs, mozzarella), complex carbohydrates (brick sheets), fibers and anti-oxidants (tomatoes) simultaneously. Its calorie intake is reasonable: 295 kcal per serving, it is suitable for overweight.

OMELET WITH COTTAGE CHEESE AND FRUITS

INGREDIENT

- 2 eggs
- 1 tbsp. (15 mL) water
- 1/4 cup (60 mL) low-sodium cottage cheese
- 1/2 cup (125 mL) drained canned fruit mingue
- icing sugar (optional)

PREPARATION

1. Whisk eggs and water in a bowl.
2. Spray an 8-inch (20 cm) nonstick skillet with cooking spray. Heat the pan over medium heat. Pour in the egg mixture. As the eggs begin to cook near the wall, using a spatula, gently scrape the cooked portions towards the center. Bend and turn the pan to allow the uncooked egg to flow into the free space.
3. When eggs are cooked on top but still wet, evenly spread the cottage cheese in the center of the omelet. Using a spoon, place a cup of fruit Macedonia on the cheese. Fold each side of the omelet towards the center and the fruit Macedonia.
4. Slide the omelet on a plate. Sprinkle with 1/4 cup of the fruit Macedonia and, if desired, sifted icing sugar.

FRENCH TOAST WITH APPLES AND MINT

INGREDIENTS

- 2 eggs, beaten lightly
- 1/8 tsp. at t. (1/2 mL) mint
- ½ cup (125 mL) milk
- ¾ cup (175 mL) applesauce
- 4 slices white bread

PREPARATION

1. In a bowl, combine eggs, milk, and mint.
2. Add the applesauce to the mixture.
3. Melt some margarine in a nonstick skillet over medium-high heat.
4. Dip the bread slices in the mixture and place it in the pan.
5. When the side of the bread facing down is brown, return the slice and cook the other side.
6. Garnish with syrup.
7. Apple and Mint French Toast, 5.0 out of 5 based on 1 rating.

CHAPTER 13
BREAKFAST RECIPES
OATMEAL AND FRUIT MUFFINS

INGREDIENTS

- 1 1/2 cup whole wheat bread flour or all-purpose
- 1 cup quick-cooking oatmeal
- 3/4 cups brown sugar whole or dark
- 2 teaspoons baking powder
- 1/2 teaspoon salt
- 1 cup sour cream 5% or 14%
- 2 teaspoons baking soda
- 1/2 cup canola oil
- 2 eggs
- 1 tablespoon vanilla extract
- 2 cups fresh or frozen fruit (blueberries, cherries, peaches, blackberries, strawberries, berries, etc.)

PREPARATION

1. Preheat the oven to 350 ° F. In a bowl, combine flour, oats, baking powder, and salt with a fork. Cut the fruit into 1 to 1.5 cm pieces if they are larger.
2. Meanwhile, mix the baking soda with the sour cream in a measuring cup of 2 cups. Allow swelling.

3. With an electric mixer, mix oil with eggs and vanilla. Add the brown sugar and mix well. Add swollen sour cream and mix gently.

4. Gradually add dry ingredients to moist ingredients. Mix gently between each addition. Add the fruits and mix with a spoon.

5. Divide the dough into muffin pans covered with paper boxes. Bake the muffins in the oven for about 20 minutes.

BLUEBERRY PANCAKES

INGREDIENTS

- 2-3 cups of flour
- 2 teaspoons baking powder
- 3/4 cup flaked oatmeal
- 1/4 cup sugar
- 1 3/4 cup milk (more or less depending on taste)
- 2 eggs
- 20 grams of melted butter
- 1 tablespoon vanilla extract
- a pinch of salt
- Blueberries at ease

INSTRUCTIONS

1. Mix the flour, baking powder, oatmeal, pinch of salt, and sugar.
2. Add milk, egg yolks, melted butter, vanilla extract.
3. Raise the egg whites to the point and add them to the mixture in an envelope.
4. Cook in a pan and add the blueberries in each pancake.
5. Serve with maple honey.

BREAKFAST WITH AVENA COPOS

INGREDIENTS:

- 250 ml of milk (can be from a cow, soy, oatmeal, rice)
- 3 heaped tablespoons of oat flakes (I buy them at Mercadona)
- 1 tablespoon honey, sugar or cinnamon
- Half grated apple
- 1 handful of raisins
- Half banana cut
- 1 handful of walnuts, date chips, figs (any dried fruit)

PREPARATION:

1. Put the milk in a saucepan with the oatmeal and simmer.
2. When it starts to boil, leave about 5 minutes (stirring so that it does not stick to you), finished those 5 minutes, let stand a few minutes with the fire off (it will be more fluffy).
3. Put in a bowl and add the sweetener that you want along with the apple, banana, and nuts.
4. you can take it both hot and cold.

NOTES:

You can take them if you want only with milk. Let's see that the important thing is to put the oatmeal flakes, and if we put more rich things, it is already a DELICIOUS AND HEALTHY BREAKFAST!

__BANANA BREAKFAST PANCAKES__

INGREDIENTS :

- ½ cup (63g.) Of wheat flour.
- ½ cup (80g.) Of flaked oatmeal.
- 2 small bananas (160g.) Mashed.
- 2 eggs (100g.).
- 1 cup (240g.) Ideal, 0% Fat, Evaporated Milk.
- 2 tablespoons (30g.) Brown sugar.
- 1 tablespoon (6g.) Of cinnamon.
- 1 teaspoon (5g.) Of butter.

PROCEDURE:

- In a bowl, combine all ingredients, except butter.
- In a pan over medium heat, place the butter and wait for it to melt.
- Pour ¼ cup of the mixture over the pan and cook until it begins to bubble.
- Turn the pancake and cook for 1 minute or until it browns on the other side.
- Serve and enjoy.

ORANGE AND RED BLUEBERRY COOKIES

INGREDIENTS:

- 4 T (360g) of oatmeal in fine flakes
- 2 T (250g without bone) dates
- 1 cheaped the vanilla powder
- 1 T (120g) dried cranberries
- 2 organic oranges (its juice and peel)
- sweet orange essence salt - optional
- 2 C mild oil (sunflower or almond) - optional

PREPARATION

1. Wash the oranges and grate them. Make the juice and reserve.
2. Crush the dates.
3. Put in the robot: oat flakes, dates, orange zest, vanilla, and a pinch of salt. Crush until it begins to stick, and dates have been chopped small.
4. Add the juice of the oranges and crush again to incorporate. (200ml at most, if you get a little less, nothing happens)
5. Now add the blueberries and mash — just a little, just enough for some to chop and others not.
6. Remove the robot and put it in a bowl.

7. Add the oil, although this is optional, if you do not have or do not want to put and the dough is sufficiently moistened so that you can form the cookies, you can skip it.

8. Make the cookies and put on the dehydrator tray. They do not need to be on teflex sheet or baking paper. I leave them as-is for the air to circulate better and be done before. Set the first hour at 52 degrees and the following at 42. They will be done in about 6 hours or so; after 4 hours, you can turn them around.

TUNA SPINACH SANDWICH

INGREDIENTS

- The quantity of ingredients is to your liking and preference.
- Integral bread
- Fresh and well-washed spinach
- Tuna in well-drained water
- A ripe but firm avocado
- Salt and pepper

INSTRUCTIONS

1. The spinach already washed and dried the short in thin strips, the finest you can.
2. What I do to achieve these strips is, I arrange several spinach leaves on top of each other, I make a small roll, and with a very sharp knife, I am cutting and thus they are excellent.
3. Avocado cut it into tiny cubes.
4. The bread is browned in a Teflon pan, on one side only.
5. Mix spinach with tuna and avocado.
6. Season the mixture with salt and pepper.
7. You put the stuffing in the bread and go.
8. Enjoy this delight.

GRILLED EGGPLANTS WITH GARLIC AND HERBS

INGREDIENTS:

- 2 eggplants
- 1 teaspoon salt
- ½ cup extra virgin olive oil
- 3 grated garlic cloves
- 2 tablespoons chopped fresh parsley
- 2 tablespoons fresh oregano
- ½ teaspoon black pepper
- ½ extra teaspoon of salt

INSTRUCTIONS

1. Cut the eggplants into 5 mm slices and generously salt each of them. Let stand 15 minutes for the salt to extract moisture and bitterness from the eggplant. Clean each slice with a paper towel to remove excess moisture and salt.
2. Preheat the grill over medium heat.
3. On a large plate, mix olive oil, garlic, parsley, oregano, pepper, and salt. Pass each eggplant slice through the mixture so that it is covered with oil.
4. Roast about 6 minutes per side until golden brown and with grill marks. If they dry out, brush with more oil.
5. Serve with a drizzle of the remaining herbal oil.

BAKED OATMEAL WITH SPICED APPLE

INGREDIENTS

- one beaten egg
- 1/2 cup of applesauce
- 1 1/2 cup of milk 1% or nonfat
- 1 tsp of vanilla
- 2 tbsp of oil
- one chopped apple
- 2 cups of oats traditional
- 1 tsp of baking powder
- 1/4 teaspoon of salt
- 1 tsp of cinnamon

INGREDIENTS (from the top)

- 2 tbsp of brown sugar
- 2 tbsp of walnuts, chopped (optional)

PREPARATION

1. Heat the oven to 375 degrees F.
2. Combine the egg, applesauce, milk, vanilla, and oil in a bowl. Enter the apple.
3. In another bowl, mix oats (rolled oats), baking powder, salt, and cinnamon. Add to liquid ingredients and mix well.
4. Pour the mixture into a ceramic baking plate and put it in the oven for 25 minutes.

168

5. Remove the bowl from the oven, sprinkle with brown sugar and nuts (optional) on top.

6. Return the bowl to the oven and cook for 3 to 4 minutes until the top is golden brown and the sugar bubbles.

7. Serve warm. Refrigerate leftovers within 2 hours.

CHICKEN AND PEAR SALAD

INGREDIENTS

- Escarole, canons or watercress
- Grilled chicken
- Pear
- Pistachios
- sweet onion (rings)
- Pink pepper
- Pink salt
- Extra virgin olive oil 3 tablespoons
- 1 teaspoon Dijon mustard in grain
- 1 teaspoon honey

INSTRUCTIONS

1. Clean and cut delicious escarole or any other green leafy vegetable such as canons, watercress to which you add a few pieces of pear cut into segments or squares.
2. Add chopped pistachios.
3. You can use any other dried fruit that you like more or that you have in the pantry: pine nuts, pecans, almonds.
4. Peel and chop onion, which gives it a spicy point always.
5. And if you dare with the vinaigrette mix, a teaspoon of Dijon mustard in grain, a

teaspoon of honey, extra virgin olive oil, lime juice and salt, and pink pepper.

6. Pink pepper is an ingredient that gives an extraordinary touch, in my opinion, and you can crush some and others you leave them whole.

7. The so-called pink pepper, in reality, is the grain of a Brazilian pepper shaker. Its flavor is very peculiar, the mixture of sweet, citrus, little spicy flavor, reminiscent of pine.

8. Finally, you add the roast chicken that you can buy well packed or remains of some homemade preparation.

SPAGHETTI WITH BROCCOLI SAUCE (BROCCOLI) PESTO TYPE

INGREDIENTS:

- 500 gr. of spaghetti or noodles (use long pasta of your choice)
- 1 broccoli (broccoli) of approx. 600 gr.
- 2 tablespoons olive oil
- ½ medium onion
- 2 cloves of garlic
- 50 gr. of walnuts
- 1 cup chicken broth or vegetable broth
- 1 tablespoon of cream or sour cream or ½ cup of cream
- 50 gr. grated Parmesan cheese
- nutmeg to your liking
- salt and black pepper to your taste
- flaked chili or cayenne pepper to your liking (optional)

PREPARATION:

1. Wash and cut into broccoli (broccoli) on florets, making sure that the size is similar to cook at the same time. Cut across at the bottom of the trunk. This will make the trunk and the flower cook at the same time. Take advantage of the trunk, which is also

172

very tasty. Simply peel it a bit and cut it into discs.

2. In a large pot with a lid, pour only two fingers of water. Add salt, mix well and introduce broccoli (broccoli). Try to place the florets with the trunk down and the flower up, since, in this way, the flower will not wilt during cooking. Cook covered over medium heat for 10 minutes or until a knife is easily inserted into the trunk.

3. Turn off the heat, drain the broccoli (broccoli) in a colander and return it to the pot.

4. While broccoli (broccoli) is cooking, cut the onion and garlic into brunoise and brown in a pan with a little olive oil until they are translucent. Turn off the heat, add the nuts and wait for the broccoli (broccoli) to be cooked.

5. Add the sautéed onion to broccoli (broccoli), and with the help of a crusher, blender, or blender, blend all the ingredients until you get a homogeneous mixture. Add chicken or vegetable broth, cream, nutmeg, salt, pepper and continue beating. Add grated Parmesan cheese and mix with the help of a spatula or wooden spoon. If you want it spicy, add some chili flakes to your liking.

6. Cover the pot and set aside until the pasta is cooked.

7. In a large pot with plenty of saltwater, cook the spaghetti or noodles following the manufacturer's instructions. Take care that you stay "al dente." Once cooked, save a ladle of spaghetti water and drain the remaining water.

8. Mix the spaghetti with the sauce and if you need more liquid, add some water that you reserved from the spaghetti.

9. Serve immediately and spread a little "Tomatina" sauce on top.

QUESADILLAS WITH PEARS

INGREDIENTS

- 4 medium wheat whole wheat tortillas
- 1 cup of cheese grated (try cheddar or Jack)
- 1 cup of diced pears (fresh or canned and drained of liquid)
- 1/2 cup of chili green or red bell finely chopped
- 2 tbsp of onion, finely chopped (scallion, white or red)

PREPARATION

1. Divide the cheese, peas, chili peppers, and onions among the tortillas, covering almost half of each tortilla.
2. Heat a pan or iron over medium heat (300 degrees in an electric pan). Place one or two folded tortillas in a hot, dry pan until the cheese melts and the tortilla is lightly browned approximately 2-4 minutes.
3. With a large spatula, gently turn the quesadillas and cook the other side until they are a little golden, 2 to 4 minutes.
4. Put away to a plate and repeat until all tortillas are hot. Cut each cooked quesadilla in half and serve.

5. Refrigerate what about within the next 2 hours.

Notes

- Put the pears in cubes on paper towels for a couple of minutes to dry completely. This will help the quesadilla not be destroyed in the process!
- Do not have pears? Try fresh apples, grapes cut in half; or even cut bananas.
- To give more flavor: add finely cut cilantro, or use "pepper jack" type cheese.

CRANBERRY QUINOA SALAD

INGREDIENTS

- 1 1/2 cups of water
- 1 cup raw quinoa, rinsed
- 1/4 cup chopped red pepper
- 1/4 cup yellow pepper, chopped
- 1 small red/purple onion, finely chopped
- 1 1/2 teaspoons curry powder
- 1/4 cup chopped fresh cilantro
- 1 lemon, juiced
- 1/4 cup toasted sliced almonds
- 1/2 cup chopped carrots
- 1/2 cup dried cranberries
- Salt and ground black pepper to taste.

INSTRUCTIONS

1. Pour the water into a saucepan and cover with a lid. Boil over high heat, then pour the quinoa, recover and continue over low heat until the water has been absorbed, 15 to 20 minutes. Transfer to a mixing bowl and chill in the refrigerator until cold.

2. Once cold, add the red pepper, yellow pepper, onion, curry powder, cilantro, lemon juice, sliced almonds, carrots, and blueberries. Season to taste with salt and pepper. Relax before serving.

WINTER FRUIT SALAD WITH LEMON AND POPPY VINAIGRETTE

INGREDIENTS

Vinaigrette

- ½ t. (125 mL) sugar
- 2 tbsp. (10 mL) onion, finely chopped
- ½ c. (2 mL) salt
- ⅓ t. (75 mL) lemon juice
- 1 C. (5 mL) Dijon mustard
- ⅔ cup (150 mL) vegetable oil
- 1 C. (15 mL) poppy seeds

Salad

- 1 large romaine lettuce apple, shredded into small pieces (about 10 t./2.5 L)
- 1 t. (250 mL) Swiss cheese, grated
- 1 t. (250 mL) cashews
- ¼ t. (50 mL) sweetened dehydrated cranberries
- 1 medium apple (1 t./250 mL)
- 1 medium pear (1 t./250 mL)

INSTRUCTIONS

1. In a blender or food processor, place sugar, onion, salt, lemon juice, and mustard; put the lid on and mix until homogeneous.

2. While the machine is running, add the net oil slowly and stably; mix until smooth and thick. Add the poppy seeds and mix for a few more seconds.

3. In a bowl, mix all the ingredients of the salad.

SALAD IN BALSAMIC TEMPEH POT, STRAWBERRIES, AND CUCUMBER

INGREDIENTS:

- 240 g. of tempeh nature
- 1/4 cup of tamari
- 1/4 cup of maple syrup
- 1/4 cup of water
- 1/4 cup of balsamic vinegar
- 1 French shallot finely chopped
- 1/3 cup of nutritional yeast
- 1 tbsp. mustard dijon
- 1 tbsp. vegetable oil table
- 1 c. olive oil
- 1/3 cup lemon juice
- 1 cup strawberries diced
- 1 cup English cucumber diced
- 2 cups red lettuce coarsely chopped
- 1/3 cup ground seeds grilled pumpkin
- Salt and pepper

PREPARATION:

1. In a cauldron filled with boiling water, cook the tempeh for ten minutes. Drain and let stand for 1 to 2 minutes. Cut the boiled tempeh block into cubes and set aside.

2. In a bowl, add tamari, maple syrup, water, balsamic vinegar, French shallot, nutritional yeast, and Dijon mustard. Mix and reserve.

3. In a skillet over medium heat, add the vegetable oil and color the cubes of tempeh. Once lightly browned, pour all the ingredients from your bowl onto the cubes, then bring to a boil by raising the temperature of the pan to medium/high. Mix from time to time until all the liquid has evaporated — Reserve in a bowl.

4. In 2 Mason jars, divide olive oil and lemon juice equitably. Salt and pepper. Assemble the pots in equal portions and steps, adding diced strawberries, English cucumber cubes, tempeh cubes, leaf lettuce leaves, and roasted pumpkin seeds.

5. Store the Mason jars in the fridge and hang them with you in your lunches, in the park, or just for a quick meal on the way home from work. Turn the pot upside down, pour it into a bowl, mix, and enjoy immediately.

LUNCH RECIPES
FISH IN TOMATO SAUCE

INGREDIENTS

- 4 frozen white fish fillets of your choice
- 2 cups cherry tomatoes cut in half
- 2 finely sliced garlic cloves
- 120 ml light chicken broth
- 60 ml of dry white wine (or use more chicken stock)
- 1/2 teaspoon salt
- 1/2 teaspoon black pepper
- 1/4 cup finely chopped fresh basil leaves (to garnish)

PREPARATION

1. Place the tomatoes, garlic, salt, and pepper in a pan over medium heat. Cook for 5 minutes or until tomatoes is soft.
2. Add chicken broth, white wine (if used), frozen fish fillets, and chopped basil. Cover and simmer 20-25 minutes, until the fish is fully cooked.
3. Finally, sprinkle with an additional handful of chopped basil and serve on a bed of rice, couscous or quinoa, if desired.

Note: Thick white fish fillets such as cod, halibut, catfish, or mahi-mahi work best for this recipe.

SEA BASS AND PEPPERS SALAD

INGREDIENTS

- Seabass is very clean: A fillet of 150 g.
- Assorted lettuces: 100 g.
- Chives: To taste
- Fresh or roasted red pepper: 1
- Cherry tomatoes To taste
- Garlic clove and parsley 1
- Leek 1
- Carrot 1
- Olive oil One tablespoon
- Salt and lemon to taste

INSTRUCTIONS

1. We put the fillet of sea bass in aluminum foil. In the mortar, chop the garlic and parsley, add 2 small teaspoons of oil and cover the fillet of sea bass with it.

2. We also put some leek and carrot strips on the sea bass fillet (the vegetable ribbons can be made with the fruit peeler) and a little salt. Now we close the foil tightly and take it to the oven at 120 ºC for 8-10 minutes. Once cooked, let it cool.

3. In a salad bowl, we put the lettuce mixture and chop the chives and pepper very finely. We add it too. Add the cherry tomatoes cut

183

SASHA TAYLOR

into quarters. Add only a small teaspoon of olive oil, salt, and lemon as a dressing and stir well and now add the fish with the vegetables that we have cooked in the oven and ready to eat.

MEXICAN BAKED BEANS AND RICE

INGREDIENTS

- 5 ml (1 teaspoon) unsalted butter
- 1 chopped yellow onion
- 3/4 cup (190 mL) basmati rice
- 5 ml (1 teaspoon) ground cumin
- 1 seeded jalapeño pepper
- 300 ml (1 1/4 cups) chicken stock
- 125 ml (1/2 cup) tomato sauce
- 3/4 cup (190 mL) canned black kidney beans
- 30 ml (2 tablespoons) finely chopped parsley
- 1 lime
- Salt and pepper, to taste

PREPARATION

1. In a saucepan, melt the butter and add the onion. Simmer.
2. Add the rice and ground cumin. Continue cooking for about 2 minutes. Add the Jalapeno pepper. Deglaze with chicken stock and season.
3. Add the tomato sauce — cover and cook over medium heat for about 12 minutes.

4. When the rice is cooked, add the black beans and parsley. Continue cooking for minutes.
5. Add lime juice, salt, pepper, and serve.

EASY BAKED SHEPHERD PIE

INGREDIENTS

- 500 grams of freshly ground duck meat
- 3 tablespoons oil or olive oil
- 1 small onion, finely chopped
- 1 tsp ready-made garlic and salt seasoning
- 1 tablespoon dry spice chimichurri
- 4 medium cooked and mashed potatoes
- 1 tablespoon full of butter
- 100 ml of milk
- 25 grams of grated Parmesan cheese
- 1 pinch of salt

PREPARATION

1. In a pan heat oil, onion, and fry.
2. Add the meat and garlic and salt seasoning.
3. Fry well until the accumulated meat water dries.
4. After the meat is fried, add enough water to cover the meat.
5. Let it cook with the pan without a lid until the water almost dries again.
6. Add the chimichurri, stir and cook until the water dries, and the meat is fried until well dried.
7. Put the meat in an ovenproof dish and set aside.

8. Prepare a mash by mixing the remaining ingredients and spread over the meat.
9. Bake for about 20 minutes or until flushed.
10. Remove and serve.

FISH IN THE HERB, GARLIC, AND TOMATO SAUCE

INGREDIENTS

- 6 teeth garlic peeled and whole
- 300 grams of halved mini onion
- 300 grams of halved pear (or cherry) tomato
- 1 packet of herbs (basil, parsley, and thyme) coarsely chopped
- 1/2 cup of olive oil
- 1 merluza fillet
- 2 cups wheat flour
- 3 egg
- 3 cups cornmeal
- Black pepper to taste
- Frying oil
- Salt to taste

PREPARATION

1. In a large baking dish, place the garlic, onion, tomato, and herbs. Mix the olive oil, salt, and pepper.
2. Wrap the fish fillets and cover them with plastic wrap.
3. Refrigerate and marinate for 1 hour.
4. Remove the fish fillets, pass in the flour, then in the eggs beaten with a little salt and last in the cornmeal. Refrigerate.

5. Put the baking sheet with the marinade in the oven, preheated to 200 ° C, and let it bake for about 20 minutes.
6. Remove the breaded fillets from the refrigerator and fry them in hot oil until golden brown.
7. Serve the fish with the sauce in the baking dish.

HOT SALAD WITH KALE AND WHITE BEANS

INGREDIENTS:

- 1 large bunch of kale well washed
- 1-2 tablespoons olive oil
- 1 stem of fresh rosemary, with the leaves removed from the stem and cut
- 1 small onion, cut
- 1 large carrot, sliced
- ½ teaspoon finely grated lemon zest
- 1 clove garlic, minced
- Salt to taste
- 2 cups cooked lima beans or other white beans plus cooking broth or 1 can (14 ounces)
- 1 cup plain parsley, cut
- Extra virgin olive oil, to spray
- Juice from ½ to small lemon, to spray (optional)

PREPARATION

1. Remove the leaves from the kale stalks. Cut into bite-sized pieces. Set aside.
2. Drain the white beans, reserving their broth. If you use canned beans, drain and wash. Set aside.
3. In a large pot, heat the oil over medium-high heat until it starts to boil. Add the rosemary,

reserving a teaspoon, let it boil for a moment, and then add the chopped onion, carrot, and lemon zest. Mix well and reduce the temperature. Cover and "sweat" the vegetables for minutes or until they are soft and the onion is a little golden, occasionally stirring to make sure they do not stick or burn.

4. Increase the temperature to medium-high. Add the cut garlic, stir and cook for 5 minutes. Add the cut greens with a good pinch of salt and sauté until they begin to wilt and soften.

5. Add ½ cup of the bean or water broth. Bring to a boil, lower the temperature for 10 to 15 minutes, or until the greens are soft and the liquid has evaporated. Put a little more broth or water if the vegetables seem very dry.

6. Mix the chopped parsley and the remaining teaspoon of rosemary, cook for 1 minute, then add the beans to the pot. Mix carefully with the greens. Try the seasoning.

7. Put off the burner and let the quinoa stand covered for 5 minutes. Serve sprinkled with a little olive oil and some lemon juice.

SCALLION SWORDFISH

INGREDIENTS

- 800 g of swordfish
- 1 lemon (medium)
- 1 dl of olive oil
- 2 Onions
- 1 dl of White Wine
- 1 c. (dessert) chopped parsley
- 4 royal gala apples
- 1 c. (soup) Butter
- 150 g chives
- Salt q.s.
- Paprika q.s.
- Salsa q.s.

PREPARATION

1. Season the swordfish slices with salt and lemon juice. Let them marinate for 30 minutes. After this time, fry them in olive oil. Add the peeled and sliced onions to half-moons and let them sauté.

2. Cool with white wine and season with a little more salt. Sprinkle with chopped parsley. Peel the apples cut them into wedges and sauté them in butter. Peel the spring onions and add them to the fruit.

3. Season with some salt and paprika. Serve the fish topped with the spring onions and accompanied with the sauteed apple and spring onions. Garnish with parsley.

JAMBALAYA RICE RECIPE (ALSO SIMPLY CALLED JAMBALAYA)

INGREDIENTS

- 2 cups of needled rice
- 200 g boneless, skinless chicken meat, diced
- 200 g of thinly diced ham
- 1 medium onion, finely chopped
- 2 cloves garlic, minced
- 4 peeled, seedless tomatoes, chopped
- 1 stalk of chopped celery
- 1/2 diced red bell pepper
- 4 teaspoon chicken or shrimp background
- 2 tbsp tomato extract
- 2 tbsp butter
- 1/2 cup chopped green onions
- QB of salt
- 350 g of clean gray shrimp
- 1 lemon
- QB of freshly ground black pepper

Homemade Cajun Seasoning to taste

- 1 tsp garlic powder
- 1 tablespoon onion powder
- 1 tsp white ground pepper
- 1 tsp ground black pepper
- 1 teaspoon dried pepperoni pepper
- 1 tablespoon dry thyme
- 1 tablespoon dried oregano

195

- 1 tbsp spicy paprika
- 1 tablespoon dried tarragon
- 1 teaspoon ground cinnamon
- 1 teaspoon chili powder
- 1 tablespoon salt
- PS; add all ingredients and process or mash in the pestle.

PREPARATION

1. Season the prawns with lemon juice, salt, and ground pepper. Let it taste for 30 minutes. Reserve
2. In a pan, melt the butter with a little olive oil and brown the chicken cubes. Reserve
3. In the pan, fat sauté the onion and garlic until it withers.
4. Add celery, peppers, and tomatoes, and sauté for 2 minutes.
5. Add the rice and sauté; Add tomato extract and chicken or shrimp background.
6. Mix well and add the homemade Cajun spice to taste; Cook for 15 minutes over low heat, covered, without stirring.
7. Add the reserved shrimp and cook another 5 minutes or until well-dried, mixing slightly.
8. Remove from heat, sprinkle with green onions and serve very hot.

CHICK CURRY (THAI CHICKEN)

INGREDIENTS

- 2 skinless, boneless chicken breasts (not too small)
- 3 tablespoons olive oil
- 1 small onion, finely chopped
- 2 cloves garlic, minced
- 3 tablespoons curry powder
- 1 teaspoon ground cinnamon
- 1 teaspoon paprika
- 1 bay leaf
- 1/2 teaspoon freshly grated ginger root
- 1 tbsp tomato extract
- 1 bottle of coconut milk
- 1/2 lemon (juice)
- 1 red bell pepper
- 1 cup pineapple (optional)

PREPARATION

1. In a bowl season the chicken cubes with salt and lemon juice and set aside.
2. Put in a pan the olive oil, garlic, onion, and saute until golden brown.
3. Then put the chicken in the pan and saute until golden brown.
4. Add pineapple (optional), curry, cinnamon, paprika, bay leaf, tomato extract, ginger, and

red pepper. Saute for a few more minutes (if necessary, add a cup of water).

5. Add coconut milk, cook for a few more minutes and serve.

FRIED BREADED LASAGNA WITH MARINARA SAUCE

INGREDIENTS

- 6 large slices of lasagna
- 1 cup of ricotta or cottage cheese
- 1 cup of mozzarella cheese
- 3 eggs
- ½ tablespoon of Italian seasoning
- 1 tablespoon of chopped parsley
- 1 clove of crushed garlic
- Salt and pepper
- ¼ cup wheat flour
- c / n breadcrumbs
- c / n vegetable oil

INSTRUCTIONS

1. Cook in a large saucepan with water before the lasagna, according to the manufacturer's instructions.
2. Place the lasagna sheets on a previously greased baking sheet.
3. Combine ricotta cheese, mozzarella cheese, 1 egg, Italian seasoning, parsley, garlic and salt, and pepper to taste in a bowl. Incorporate all ingredients very well.

199

4. Distribute the previous mixture on each of the lasagna sheets and roll very well by pressing the filling.

5. To breach, pass each lasagna roll through bowls of flour, bowl with 2 beaten eggs, and to finish the dish with the breadcrumbs. Then enter the freezer for 30 minutes.

6. Heat plenty of oil in a deep pan. Introduce the lasagna rolls one by one and fry for 2 to 3 minutes. Place on the paper towel to remove excess oil.

7. Cut lasagna rolls in half and serve on a marinara sauce base.

Marinara sauce:

- In a medium saucepan heat 2 tablespoons of oil, add 1 finely chopped onion and 1 clove of crushed garlic and brown for 5 minutes.

- Stir with a wooden spoon to prevent burning. Add 2 cups of chopped tomato, 2 tablespoons of tomato paste, and 2 tablespoons of chopped fresh basil, ½ tablespoon of ground black pepper, 1 teaspoon of ground oregano and ½ tablespoon of salt.

- Cook until the sauce boils. Put it on low heat and continue cooking for 20 minutes or until the sauce acquires a thick consistency.

BAKED MUSHROOMS WITH PUMPKIN AND CHIPOTLE POLENTA

INGREDIENTS

- 900 g mix of mushrooms, such as maitake, jasmine ear and black shimeji - coarsely chopped - thinly sliced porcini crimini mushrooms - and coarsely chopped shiitakessem stalks
- About 1/3 cup of extra virgin olive oil
- 1 garlic head, crushed cloves
- A small handful of sage, finely chopped or sliced
- Sea salt and freshly ground black pepper.
- 1 cup cooked pumpkin puree
- 3 cups chicken broth
- Nutmeg, freshly grated
- 1 chipotle adobo sauce, seedless and finely chopped, plus a small spoon of adobo sauce
- 1 cup quick-cooking polenta
- 2 tbsp butter
- 2 tbsp honey
- Roasted seeds for decoration
- Chives, minced, for decoration

PREPARATION

1. Preheat the oven to 220 °C.
2. Mix the mushrooms with extra virgin olive oil, garlic, brine, salt, and pepper and bake for 25 minutes.
3. Meanwhile, in a small pan, put it pumpkin puree over medium heat, along with some chicken broth to dilute.
4. Season with salt, pepper, and nutmeg.
5. In another pan, put the remaining stock and bring to a boil, then add the chipotle, adobo sauce, polenta and mix using a wire whisk. Continue beating the polenta until the sides are far from the pan walls, then add the butter, honey, and beat again.
6. Combine pumpkin and polenta and serve in individual shallow bowls.
7. Top with roasted mushrooms and Siva with roasted seeds and chives for garnish.

DINNER RECIPES
MEAT AND KIDNEY PIE

INGREDIENTS

- 500 g beef (diced)
- 225 g kidneys (cow or veal, heavy clean and cut)
- 1 onion (chopped)
- 150 g mushrooms (clean and sliced)
- 250 ml beef broth
- 2 tbsp. tomato paste (optional)
- 1 tbsp. cornstarch
- 250 g puff pastry (or broken dough)
- 1 egg (beaten)
- 1 tsp. salt
- 1 tsp. pepper (ground black pepper)
- 3 tbsp. oil
- Water (to dissolve cornstarch)

INSTRUCTIONS

1. Heat the oil in a casserole and brown the beef. We take it out and reserve it.
2. In the same oil, we fry the onion until it softens.
3. Add the kidneys, tomato paste, if used, mushrooms, and broth.
4. Cover the casserole and lower the heat when the sauce begins to boil, letting it

simmer until the meat is tender about 30 minutes.

5. When it's almost done, we can start heating the oven at 180º C.

6. Mix the cornstarch with a little water and add it to the casserole where the meat and kidneys are being cooked, mixing with the sauce, season with salt and pepper, letting the stew cook 5 more minutes, until the sauce thickens.

7. We pass the meat and kidneys with their sauce to a baking dish.

8. We stretch the dough enough to cover the source as a cover. We moisten the edge of the fountain with water and press the dough against the edge to seal it.

9. We make a cut in the middle so that the steam can escape, and we paint the dough with a beaten egg.

10. We put the meat and kidney pie in the oven and let it be done for 30 minutes, or until the dough that covers the cake is browned.

11. We serve the cake very hot, almost as soon as it comes out of the oven so that the steam does not soften the dough.

CAULIFLOWER AND PUMPKIN CASSEROLE

INGREDIENTS

- 2 tbsp. olive oil
- 1/4 medium yellow onion, minced
- 6 cups chopped forage kale into small pieces (about 140 g)
- 1 little clove garlic, minced
- Salt and freshly ground black pepper
- 1/2 cup low sodium chicken broth
- 2 cups of 1.5 cm diced pumpkin (about 230 g)
- 2 cups of 1.5 cm diced zucchini (about 230 g)
- 2 tbsp. mayonnaise
- 3 cups frozen, thawed brown rice
- 1 cup grated Swiss cheese
- 1/3 cup grated Parmesan
- 1 cup panko flour
- 1 large beaten egg
- Cooking spray

PREPARATION

1. Preheat oven to 200 ° C. Heats the oil in a large nonstick skillet over medium heat. Add onions and cook, occasionally stirring, until browned and tender (about 5 minutes). Add the cabbage, garlic, and 1/2

teaspoon salt and 1/2 teaspoon pepper and cook until the cabbage is light (about 2 minutes).

2. Add the stock and continue to cook until the cabbage withers, and most of the stock evaporates (about 5 minutes). Add squash, zucchini, and 1/2 teaspoon salt and mix well. Continue cooking until the pumpkin begins to soften (about 8 minutes). Remove from heat and add mayonnaise.

3. In a bowl, combine cooked vegetables, brown rice, cheese, 1/2 cup flour, and large egg and mix well. Spray a 2-liter casserole with cooking spray. Spread the mixture across the bottom of the pan and cover with the remaining flour, 1/4 teaspoon salt and a few pinches of pepper. Bake until the squash and zucchini are tender and the top golden and crispy (about 35 minutes). Serve hot.

Advance Preparation Tip: Freeze the casserole for up to 2 weeks. Cover with aluminum foil and heat at 180 ° C until warm (35 to 45 minutes).

THAI BEEF SALAD TEARS OF THE TIGER

INGREDIENTS

- 800 g of beef tenderloin
  For the marinade:
- 2 tablespoons of soy sauce
- 1 tablespoon soup of honey
- 1 pinch of the pepper mill
  For the sauce:
- 1 small bunch of fresh coriander
- 1 small bouquet of mint
- 3 tablespoons soup of fish sauce
- lemon green
- 1 clove of garlic
- tablespoons soup of sugar palm (or brown sugar)
- 1 bird pepper or ten drops of Tabasco
- 1 small glass of raw Thai rice to make grilled rice powder
- 200 g of arugula or young shoots of salad

PREPARATION

1. Cut the beef tenderloin into strips and put it in a container. Sprinkle with 2 tablespoons soy sauce, 1 tablespoon honey, and pepper. Although soak thoroughly and let marinate 1 hour at room temperature.

2. Meanwhile, prepare the roasted rice powder. Pour a glass of Thai rice into an anti-adhesive pan. Dry color the rice, constantly stirring to avoid burning. When it has a lovely color, get rid of it on a plate and let it cool.

3. When it has cooled, reduce it to powder by mixing it with the robot.

4. Wash and finely chop mint and coriander. Put in a container and add lime juice, chopped garlic clove, 3 tablespoons Nuoc mam, 3 tablespoons brown sugar, 3 tablespoons water, 1 tablespoon sauce soy, and a dozen drops of Tabasco. Mix well and let stand the time that the sugar melts and the flavors mix.

5. Place a bed of salad on a dish. Cook the beef strips put them on the salad. Sprinkle with the spoonful of sauce and roasted rice powder. To be served as is or with a Thai cooked white rice scented.

STUFFED APPLES WITH SHRIMP

INGREDIENTS

- 6 medium apples
- 1 lemon juice
- 2 tablespoons butter

Filling:

- 300 gr of shrimp
- 1 onion minced
- ½ cup chopped parsley
- 2 tbsp flour
- 1 can of cream/cream
- 100 gr of curd
- 1 tablespoon butter
- 1 tbsp pepper sauce
- Salt to taste

PREPARATION

1. Cut a cap from each apple, remove the seeds a little from the pulp on the sides, and put the pulp in the bottom, but leaving a cavity.
2. Pass a little lemon and some butter on the apples, bake them in the oven. Remove from oven, let cool and bring to freeze.
3. Prepare the shrimp sauce in a pan by mixing the butter with the flour, onion, parsley, and pepper sauce.

4. Then add the prawn shrimp to the sauce. When boiling, mix the cream cheese and sour cream.
5. Stuff each apple. Serve hot or cold, as you prefer.

A QUICK RECIPE OF GRILLED CHICKEN SALAD WITH ORANGES

INGREDIENTS:

- 75 ml (1/3 cup) orange juice
- 30 ml (2 tablespoons) lemon juice
- 45 ml (3 tablespoons) of extra virgin olive oil
- 15 ml (1 tablespoon) Dijon mustard
- 2 cloves of garlic, chopped
- 1 ml (1/4 teaspoon) salt, or as you like
- Freshly ground pepper to your taste
- 1 lb. (450 g) skinless chicken breast, trimmed
- 25 g (1/4 cup) pistachio or flaked almonds, toasted
- 600 g (8c / 5 oz) of mesclun, rinsed and dried
- 75 g (1/2 cup) minced red onion
- 2 medium oranges, peeled, quartered and sliced

PREPARATION:

1. Place the orange juice, lemon juice, oil, mustard, garlic, salt, and pepper in a small bowl or jar with an airtight lid; whip or shake to mix. Reserve 75 milliliters (1/3 cup) of this salad vinaigrette and 45 milliliters (three tablespoons) for basting.

211

2. Place the rest of the vinaigrette in a shallow glass dish or resealable plastic bag. Add the chicken and turn it over to coat. Cover or close and marinate in the refrigerator for at least 20 minutes or up to two hours.

3. Preheat the barbecue over medium heat. Lightly oil the grill by rubbing it with a crumpled paper towel soaked in oil (use the tongs to hold the paper towel). Remove the chicken from the marinade and discard the marinade. Grill the chicken 10 to 15 centimeters (four to six inches) from the heat source, basting the cooked sides with the basting vinaigrette until it is no longer pink in the center, and Instant-read thermometer inserted in the thickest part records 75 ° C (170 ° F), four to six minutes on each side. Transfer the chicken to a cutting board and let it rest for five minutes.

4. Meanwhile, grill almonds (or pistachios) in a small, dry pan on medium-low heat, stirring constantly, until lightly browned, about two to three minutes. Transfer them to a bowl and let them cool.

5. Place the salad and onion mixture in a large bowl. Mix with the vinaigrette reserved for the salad. Divide the salad into four plates. Slice chicken and spread on salads. Sprinkle orange slices on top and sprinkle with pistachios (or almonds).

RED CURRY WITH VEGETABLE

INGREDIENTS

- 600 g sweet potatoes
- 200 g canned chickpeas
- 2 leek whites
- 2 tomatoes
- 100 g of spinach shoots
- 40 cl of coconut milk
- 1 jar of Greek yogurt
- 1 lime
- 3 cm fresh ginger
- 1 small bunch of coriander
- 1/2 red onion
- 2 cloves garlic
- 4 tbsp. red curry paste
- Salt

PREPARATION

1. Peel the sweet potatoes and cut them into pieces. Clean the leek whites and cut them into slices. Peel and seed the tomatoes.
2. Mix the Greek yogurt with a drizzle of lime juice, chopped onion, salt, and half of the coriander leaves.
3. In a frying pan, heat 15 cl of coconut milk until it reduces and forms a multitude of

small bubbles. Brown curry paste with chopped ginger and garlic.

4. Add vegetables, drained chickpeas, remaining coconut milk, and salt. Cook for 20 min covered, then 5 min without lid for the sauce to thicken.

5. When serving, add spinach sprouts and remaining coriander. Serve with the yogurt sauce.

BAKED TURKEY BREAST WITH CRANBERRY SAUCE

INGREDIENTS

- 2 kilos of whole turkey breast
- 1 tablespoon olive oil
- 1/4 cup onion
- 2 cloves of garlic
- Thyme
- Poultry seasonings
- You saved
- Coarse-grained salt
- 2 butter spoons
- 1/4 cup minced echallot
- 1/4 cup chopped onion
- 1 clove garlic
- 2 tablespoons flour
- 1 1/2 cups of blueberries
- 2 cups apple cider
- 2 tablespoons maple honey
- Peppers

PREPARATION

1. Grind in the blender ¼ cup onion, 2 garlic with herbs. Add 1 tablespoon of oil and spread the breast with this.
2. Put in the baking tray, add a cup of citron and bake at 350 Fahrenheit (180 ° C) to

215

have a thermometer record 165 Fahrenheit (75 ° C) inside, about an hour, add ½ cup of water if necessary.

3. Bring the citron to a boil, add the blueberries, and leave a few minutes. In the butter (2 tablespoons), acitronar the onion (1/4 cup), echallot, and garlic (1 clove).

4. Add the flour to the onion and echallot and leave a few minutes. Add the citron, cranberries, and honey and leave on low heat. Season with salt and pepper, let the blueberries are soft, go to the processor, and if you want to strain.

5. Return to the fire and let it thicken slightly.

6. Slice the thin turkey breast and serve with the blueberry sauce.

PARSNIP SOUP, PEAR WITH SMOKED NUTS

INGREDIENTS

For the soup:

500g of chopped parsnips, 1 tablespoon of olive oil, 4 sprigs of thyme, salt and pepper, 1 chopped onion, 1 tablespoon of margarine, 2 peeled and chopped pears, 800 ml of vegetable stock, 600 ml of milk, 75 g of crushed California Nuts until a flour texture is achieved

For smoked nuts:

2 tsp of maple syrup, 1 teaspoon of smoked paprika, 2 teaspoons of soy sauce, 50 g of California Nuts, 1 tablespoon of chopped scallions and a dash of olive oil to decorate

INSTRUCTION

1. Preheat the oven to 180ºC. Place the parsnips on a baking sheet and squirt olive oil. Season with thyme, pepper, and salt mix well and bake for 25-30 minutes until golden brown.
2. Meanwhile, prepare smoked nuts. Mix the maple syrup, paprika, and soy sauce, spread on the nuts, and mix well. Position the nuts on a baking sheet and bake them for 8-10 minutes. Remove from the oven and let cool.

3. Next, sauté the onion with the margarine over medium heat. Add the pear and continue skipping for 8-10 more minutes.

4. Add the parsnip and the vegetable stock to the pan and continue cooking for 15 more minutes with the lid on. Add the milk and stir until creamy. Add the crushed nuts and season to taste.

5. Place the soup in bowls and decorate with smoked nuts and chopped chives. Add a dash of olive oil and serve.

MOROCCAN STYLE CHICKPEA SOUP

INGREDIENTS

- 4 ripe tomatoes, chopped
- 250 g of cooked chickpeas.
- 1 chopped onion.
- 1 branch of chopped celery.
- 2 chicken thighs
- 2 tablespoons chopped fresh cilantro.
- 2 tablespoons chopped fresh parsley.
- 1 tablespoon turmeric.
- 1 tablespoon of cinnamon coffee
- 2 tablespoons grated fresh ginger coffee.
- A few strands of saffron.
- 4 tablespoons olive oil.
- A nip of sea salt and black pepper.
- Half grated zucchini with spiralizer (noodle substitute).

PREPARATION

1. We marinate chicken thighs with cinnamon and turmeric.
2. In a deep casserole, sauté chicken thighs in olive oil and brown them for about 3-4 minutes.
3. Then add the chopped onion and grated ginger. We stir well.

4. Add the celery, parsley, and cilantro. Saute the whole over medium heat for a few minutes.
5. Next, we remove the chicken thighs and reserve them.
6. Add the chopped tomatoes and a tablespoon of olive oil to the casserole.
7. In a cup of hot water, we soak the saffron threads. Then add the saffron along with the water to the casserole.
8. Then add the chicken and three more cups of hot water.
9. Add the salt and pepper.
10. Cover the casserole and let the whole cook for half an hour, stirring occasionally.
11. Remove the chicken from the casserole, remove the bones, and add the shredded meat back to the casserole.
12. Finally, we incorporate the chickpeas.
13. Prepare the "spaghetti" zucchini with the spiralizer (noodle substitutes).
14. We serve the soup in bowls, incorporating the zucchini spaghetti on top.

TUSCAN SOUP OF CHARD AND WHITE BEANS

INGREDIENTS

- 2 slices of finely chopped bacon
- 1 chopped onion
- 1 clove garlic minced
- 1/4 c. nutmeg (optional)
- 1/8 c. hot pepper flakes (optional)
- 6-7 cups chicken broth, or more as needed
- 1 can (540 ml) of white beans, drained and rinsed
- 2 tbsp. sun-dried tomatoes, chopped
- 1 piece of Parmesan rind (about 1/2 cup)
- 1 bunch of chard red or white
- 1/4 cup small pasta for soup
- 5 large sliced sage leaves
- 5 fresh basil leaves, chopped (optional)
- 1 C. grated Parmesan cheese, divided (optional)
- 1 C. extra virgin olive oil, divided (optional)

PREPARATION

1. In a big saucepan over medium heat, brown bacon with onion, garlic, nutmeg, and pepper flakes for 5 minutes. Add chicken broth and beans. Bring to a boil. Stir in the dried tomatoes and Parmesan rind. Reduce heat and cook for 10 minutes.

221

2. Meanwhile, seed Swiss chard and slice stems into 3/4 inch lengths. Cut the leaves into 1-inch wide strips. Add the stems and pasta to the soup. Reserve the leaves for later. Reduce to low heat and simmer gently until the pasta is tender about 10 minutes. Add Swiss chard and basil leaves and simmer for 3-4 minutes.

3. Transfer soup to bowls sprinkles with parmesan and drizzle with olive oil, if desired.

DESSERTS AND SWEETS
OATMEAL AND BERRY MUFFINS

INGREDIENTS

- 1 cup (250 mL) non-blanched all-purpose flour
- ½ cup (125 mL) quick-cooking oatmeal 1/2 cup
- (160 mL) stuffed brown sugar
- 1/2 tbsp (1/2 cup) tea) baking soda
- 2 eggs
- 125 ml (1/2 cup) applesauce
- 60 ml (1/4 cup)
- orange canola oil 1, grated rind only
- 1 lemon, grated rind
- 15 ml (1 tbsp) lemon juice
- 180 ml (3/4 cup) fresh raspberries (see note)
- 180 ml (3/4 cup) fresh or blueberries (or blackberries)

PREPARATION

1. Put the grill at the center of the oven. Preheat oven to 180 ° C (350 ° F). Line 12 muffin cups with paper or silicone trays.
2. In a bowl, combine flour, oatmeal, brown sugar, and baking soda. Book.

3. In a big bowl, whisk together eggs, applesauce, oil, citrus zest, and lemon juice. Add the dry ingredients to the wooden spoon. Add the berries and mix gently.
4. Spread the mixture in the boxes. Sprinkle top with pistachio muffins. Bake for 20 to 22 minutes or until a toothpick inserted in the center of a muffin comes out clean. Let cool.

CRUNCHY BLUEBERRY AND APPLES

INGREDIENTS

Crunchy

- 1 cup (1¼ cup) quick-cooking oatmeal
- ¼ cup (60 mL) brown sugar
- ¼ cup (60 mL) unbleached all-purpose flour
- 90 ml (6 tablespoons) melted margarine

Garnish

- 125 ml (½ cup) brown sugar
- 20 ml (4 teaspoons) cornstarch
- 1 liter (4 cups) fresh or frozen blueberries (not thawed)
- 500 ml (2 cups) grated apples
- 1 Tbsp.
- (15 mL) melted margarine 15 mL (1 tablespoon) lemon juice

PREPARATION

1. Put the grill at the center of the oven. Preheat oven to 180 ° C (350 ° F).
2. In a bowl, mix dry ingredients. Add the margarine and mix until the mixture is just moistened. Book.
3. In a 20-cm (8-inch) square baking pan, combine brown sugar and cornstarch. Add the fruits, margarine, lemon juice, and mix

well. Cover with crisp and bake between 55 minutes and 1 hour, or until the crisp is golden brown. Serve warm or cold.

RASPBERRY FEAST MERINGUE WITH CREAM DIPLOMAT

INGREDIENTS

Preparation of meringue

- 2 egg whites
- 1/2 cup caster sugar
- 1/4 tsp. vanilla extract
- 1/4 cup crumbled barley sugar

Raspberry mousse preparation

- 1 cup frozen raspberries
- 1/4 cup water
- 2 tbsp. Raspberry Jell-O Powder with No Added Sugar
- 1 1/2 cup Cool Whip
- 1 bowl fresh raspberries

PREPARATION

1. To make the meringue, preheat the oven to 350 o F (175 o C) and line a baking sheet with parchment paper.
2. In a blender or bowl, whisk egg whites until the foam is obtained. Gently add the sugar while whisking until you get firm, shiny picks. Stir in vanilla extract and crumbled barley sugar.

3. Shape the meringues on the coated cookie sheet and place in the preheated oven. Turn off the oven and wait 2 hours. Do not open the oven. Once the meringues are dry, break the meringues into small bites.
4. To make the mousse, put frozen raspberries and water in a small saucepan. Heat until raspberries melt and are tender. Put these raspberries in a blender. Add the Jell-O powder and mix. Once the raspberries have completely cooled, incorporate the Cool Whip.
5. To shape the raspberry, place in balloon glasses for individual portions or in a large cake pan first a layer of raspberry mousse, then a layer of meringue, then fresh raspberries. Repeat the layers. Refrigerate for a few hours before serving.

CHEESECAKE MOUSSE WITH RASPBERRIES

INGREDIENTS

- 1 cup light lemonade filling
- 1 can 8 oz cream cheese at room temperature
- 3/4 cup SPLENDA no-calorie sweetener pellets
- 1 tbsp. at t. of lemon zest
- 1 tbsp. at t. vanilla extract
- 1 cup fresh or frozen raspberries

PREPARATION

1. Beat the cream cheese until it is sparkling; add 1/2 cup SPLENDA® Granules and mix until melted. Stir in lemon zest and vanilla.
2. Reserve some raspberries for decoration. Crush the rest of the raspberries with a fork and mix them with 1/4 cup SPLENDA pellets until they are melted.
3. Lightly add the lump and cheese filling, and then gently but quickly add crushed raspberries. Share this mousse in 6 ramekins with a spoon and keep in the refrigerator until tasting.
4. Garnish mousses with reserved raspberries and garnish with fresh mint before serving.

ALMOND MERINGUE COOKIES

INGREDIENTS

- 2 egg whites or 4 tbsp. pasteurized egg whites (at room temperature)
- 1 Tbsp. tartar cream
- ½ tsp.
- ½ teaspoon almond extract vanilla extract
- ½ cup white sugar

PREPARATION

1. Preheat the oven to 300F.
2. Whisk the egg whites with the cream of tartar until the volume has doubled. Add other ingredients and whip until peaks form.
3. Using two teaspoons, drop a spoonful of meringue onto parchment paper with the back of the other spoon.
4. Bake at 300F for about 25 minutes or until the meringues are crisp. Place in an airtight container.

FRESH CRANBERRY PIE

INGREDIENTS

- 1 ½ cup crumbled Graham crackers
- ¼ cup salt-free chopped pecans
- 1 ¾ cup Splenda Sweetener
- ½ cup non-hydrogenated salt-free margarine
- 1 ½ cup freshly picked cranberries
- 2 egg whites
- 1 tbsp. thawed apple juice concentrate
- 1 tbsp. vanilla extract
- 1 liter Cool Whip Whipped Topping, thawed

Cranberry Frosting:

- ¼ cup Splenda Sweetener
- ¼ cup caster sugar
- 1 Tbsp. cornstarch
- ¾ cup fresh cranberries
- ¾ cup of water

PREPARATION

1. Preheat oven to 375 ° F (190 ° C).
2. Mix crumbled crackers, pecans, and ¾ cup of Splenda. Add the margarine, mix well, and arrange on a hinged mold pressing on the bottom and the sides. Bake dough for 6 minutes or until slightly browned. Let cool.

3. Mix the cranberries with 1 cup of Splenda. Let stand for 5 minutes. Add the egg whites, apple juice, and vanilla. Beat at low speed until foamy, and then beat at high speed for 5 to 8 minutes until mixture is firm.

4. Stir in the whipped topping in the cranberry mixture. Pour the mixture over the pre-cooked dough. Refrigerate at least 4 hours until the mixture is firm.

5. To make the icing, mix the sugar, Splenda, and cornstarch in a saucepan. Stir in cranberries and water. Cook, stirring until bubbles appear. Continue cooking, occasionally stirring until cranberry skin comes off. Use the mixture at room temperature. Do not refrigerate: the sauce may crystallize and become opaque.

6. Remove the tart from the pan and arrange on a serving platter; using a spoon, coat with icing.

ENTRIES AND SNACKS
EGGPLANT AND CHICKPEA BITES

INGREDIENTS

- 3 large aubergines cut in half (make a few cuts in the flesh with a knife) Spray
- oil
- 2 large cloves garlic, peeled and deglazed
- 2 tbsp. coriander powder
- 2 tbsp. cumin seeds
- 400 g canned chickpeas, rinsed and drained
- 2 Tbsp. chickpea flour
- Zest and juice of 1/2 lemon
- 1/2 lemon quartered for serving
- 3 tbsp. tablespoon of polenta

PREPARATION

1. Heat the oven to 200ºC (180ºC rotating heat, gas level 6). Spray the eggplant halves generously with oil and place them on the meat side up on a baking sheet. Sprinkle with coriander and cumin seeds, and then place the cloves of garlic on the plate. Season and roast for 40 minutes until the flesh of eggplant is completely tender. Reserve and let cool a little.
2. Scrape the flesh of the eggplant in a bowl with a spatula and throw the skins in the

233

compost. Thoroughly scrape and make sure to incorporate spices and crushed roasted garlic. Add chickpeas, chickpea flour, zest, and lemon juice. Crush roughly and mix well, check to season. Do not worry if the mixture seems a bit soft - it will firm up in the fridge.

3. Form about twenty pellets and place them on a baking sheet covered with parchment paper. Let stand in the fridge for at least 30 minutes.

4. Preheat oven to 180ºC (rotating heat 160ºC, gas level 4). Remove the meatballs from the fridge and coat them by rolling them in the polenta. Place them back on the baking sheet and spray a little oil on each. Roast for 20 minutes until golden and crisp. Serve with lemon wedges. You can also serve these dumplings with a spicy yogurt dip with harissa, this delicious but spicy mashed paste of hot peppers and spices from the Maghreb.

POPCORN WITH SUGAR AND SPICE

INGREDIENTS

- 8 cups hot popcorn
- 2 tablespoons unsalted butter
- 2 tablespoons sugar
- 1/2 teaspoon cinnamon
- 1/4 teaspoon nutmeg

PREPARATION

1. Popping the corn; put aside.
2. Heat the butter, sugar, cinnamon, and nutmeg in the microwave or saucepan over a range fire until the butter is melted and the sugar dissolved.
3. Be careful not to burn the butter.
4. Sprinkle the corn with the spicy butter, mix well.
5. Serve immediately for optimal flavor.

BABA GHANOUJ

INGREDIENTS

- 1 large aubergine, cut in half lengthwise
- 1 head of garlic, unpeeled
- 30 ml (2 tablespoons) of olive oil
- Lemon juice to taste

PREPARATION

1. Put the grill at the center of the oven. Preheat the oven to 350 ° F. Line a baking sheet with parchment paper.
2. Place the eggplant on the plate, skin side up. Roast until the meat is very tender and detaches easily from the skin, about 1 hour depending on the size of the eggplant. Let cool.
3. Meanwhile, cut the tip of the garlic cloves. Place the garlic cloves in a square of aluminum foil. Fold the edges of the sheet and fold together to form a tightly wrapped foil. Roast with the eggplant until tender, about 20 minutes. Let cool. Purée the pods with a garlic press.
4. With a spoon, scoop out the flesh of the eggplant and place it in the bowl of a food processor. Add the garlic puree, the oil, and the lemon juice. Stir until purée is smooth and pepper.
5. Serve with mini pita bread.

BAKED PITA CHIPS

INGREDIENTS

- 3 pita loaves (6 inches)
- 3 tablespoons olive oil
- Chili powder

PREPARATION

1. Separate each bread in half with scissors, to obtain 6 round pieces. Cut each piece into eight points. Brush each with olive oil and sprinkle with chili powder. Bake at 350 degrees F for about 15 minutes until crisp.

MIXES OF SNACKS

INGREDIENTS

- 6 c. margarine
- 2 tbsp. Worcestershire sauce
- 1 ½ tbsp. spice salt
- ¾ c. garlic powder
- ½ tsp. onion powder
- 3 cups Crispix
- 3 cups Cheerios
- 3 cups corn flakes
- 1 cup Kix
- 1 cup pretzels
- 1 cup broken bagel chips into 1-inch pieces

PREPARATION

1. Preheat the oven to 250F (120C)
2. Melt the margarine in a large roasting pan. Stir in the seasoning. Gradually add the ingredients remaining by mixing so that the coating is uniform.
3. Cook 1 hour, stirring every 15 minutes. Spread on paper towels to let cool. Store in a tightly-closed container.

HERBAL CREAM CHEESE TARTINES

INGREDIENTS

- 20 regular round melba crackers
- 1 clove garlic, halved
- 1 cup cream cheese spread
- ¼ cup chopped herbs such as chives, dill, parsley, tarragon or thyme
- 2 tbsp. minced French shallot or onion
- ½ tsp. black pepper
- 2 tbsp. tablespoons water

PREPARATION

1. In a medium-sized bowl, combine the cream cheese, herbs, shallot, pepper, and water with a hand blender.
2. Rub the crackers with the cut side of the garlic clove.
3. Serve the cream cheese with the rusks.

SPICY CRAB DIP

INGREDIENTS

- 1 can of 8 oz softened cream cheese
- 1 tbsp. to s. finely chopped onions
- 1 tbsp. at t. lemon juice
- 2 tbsp. at t. Worcestershire sauce
- 1/8 tsp. at t. black
- pepper Cayenne pepper to taste
- 2 tbsp. to s. of milk or non-fortified rice drink
- 1 can of 6 oz of crabmeat

PREPARATION

1. Preheat the oven to 375 ° F (190 ° C).
2. Pour the cream cheese into a bowl. Add the onions, lemon juice, Worcestershire sauce, black pepper, and cayenne pepper. Mix well. Stir in the milk/rice drink. Add the crabmeat and mix until you obtain a homogeneous mixture.
3. Pour the mixture into a baking dish. Cook without covering for 15 minutes or until bubbles appear. Serve hot with low-sodium crackers or triangle cut pita bread. OR
4. Microwave until bubbles appear, about 4 minutes, stirring every 1 to 2 minutes.

Lightning Source UK Ltd.
Milton Keynes UK
UKHW022046160223
417160UK00003B/527